DELIBERATE PRACTICE IN
INTERPERSONAL
PSYCHOTHERAPY

Essentials of Deliberate Practice Series
Tony Rousmaniere and Alexandre Vaz, Series Editors

Deliberate Practice in Child and Adolescent Psychotherapy
Jordan Bate, Tracy A. Prout, Tony Rousmaniere, and
Alexandre Vaz

Deliberate Practice in Cognitive Behavioral Therapy
James F. Boswell and Michael J. Constantino

Deliberate Practice in Dialectical Behavior Therapy
Tali Boritz, Shelley McMain, Alexandre Vaz, and
Tony Rousmaniere

Deliberate Practice in Emotion-Focused Therapy
Rhonda N. Goldman, Alexandre Vaz, and Tony Rousmaniere

Deliberate Practice in Interpersonal Psychotherapy
Olga Belik, Jessica M. Schultz, Scott Fairhurst, Scott Stuart,
Alexandre Vaz, and Tony Rousmaniere

Deliberate Practice in Motivational Interviewing
Jennifer K. Manuel, Denise Ernst, Alexandre Vaz, and
Tony Rousmaniere

Deliberate Practice in Multicultural Therapy
Jordan Harris, Joel Jin, Sophia Hoffman, Selina Phan,
Tracy A. Prout, Tony Rousmaniere, and Alexandre Vaz

Deliberate Practice in Psychedelic-Assisted Therapy
Shannon Dames, Andrew Penn, Monnica Williams,
Joseph A. Zamaria, Tony Rousmaniere, and Alexandre Vaz

Deliberate Practice in Psychodynamic Psychotherapy
Hanna Levenson, Volney Gay, and Jeffrey L. Binder

Deliberate Practice in Rational Emotive Behavior Therapy
Mark D. Terjesen, Kristene A. Doyle, Raymond A. DiGiuseppe,
Alexandre Vaz, and Tony Rousmaniere

Deliberate Practice in Schema Therapy
Wendy T. Behary, Joan M. Farrell, Alexandre Vaz, and
Tony Rousmaniere

Deliberate Practice in Systemic Family Therapy
Adrian J. Blow, Ryan B. Seedall, Debra L. Miller,
Tony Rousmaniere, and Alexandre Vaz

ESSENTIALS OF DELIBERATE PRACTICE SERIES
TONY ROUSMANIERE AND ALEXANDRE VAZ, SERIES EDITORS

DELIBERATE PRACTICE IN
INTERPERSONAL PSYCHOTHERAPY

OLGA BELIK

JESSICA M. SCHULTZ

SCOTT FAIRHURST

SCOTT STUART

ALEXANDRE VAZ

TONY ROUSMANIERE

AMERICAN PSYCHOLOGICAL ASSOCIATION

Published by
American Psychological Association
750 First Street, NE
Washington, DC 20002
https://www.apa.org

Order Department
https://www.apa.org/pubs/books
order@apa.org

Typeset in Cera Pro by Circle Graphics, Inc., Reisterstown, MD

Printer: Gasch Printing, Odenton, MD
Cover Designer: Mark Karis

Library of Congress Cataloging-in-Publication Data

Names: Belik, Olga, author. | American Psychological Association, publisher.
Title: Deliberate practice in interpersonal psychotherapy / authored by
  Olga Belik, Jessica M. Schultz, Scott Fairhurst, Scott Stuart, Alexandre Vaz,
  and Tony Rousmaniere.
Other titles: Essentials of deliberate practice series
Description: Washington, DC : American Psychological Association, [2025] |
  Series: Essentials of deliberate practice series | Includes bibliographical
  references and index.
Identifiers: LCCN 2024020570 (print) | LCCN 2024020571 (ebook) |
  ISBN 9781433840463 (paperback) | ISBN 9781433840470 (ebook)
Subjects: MESH: Interpersonal Psychotherapy--education | Role Playing |
  Problems and Exercises | BISAC: PSYCHOLOGY / Education & Training |
  PSYCHOLOGY / Clinical Psychology
Classification: LCC RC489.P7 (print) | LCC RC489.P7 (ebook) | NLM WM 18.2 |
  DDC 616.89/1523--dc23/eng/20241008
LC record available at https://lccn.loc.gov/2024020570
LC ebook record available at https://lccn.loc.gov/2024020571

https://doi.org/10.1037/0000426-000

Printed in the United States of America

10 9 8 7 6 5 4 3 2 1

To my wife, Deb, and my twin daughters, Nina and Rose. With deep gratitude for your light and love. To my brilliant coauthors and entire interpersonal psychotherapy community, with appreciation for your contributions to my personal and professional growth and for the strong interpersonal commitment that you hold for everyone in your life. May this book further our intentions and efforts to establish and maintain genuine, transparent, and healthy connections with each other in this world.

—Olga Belik

To my family. With deep gratitude to the interpersonal psychotherapy community, and especially my wise, kind, generous coauthors. And with reverence for the courage of clients seeking care and therapists providing it. It is my deep hope that this book may contribute to recovery, healing, and growth.

—Jessica M. Schultz

I would like to acknowledge my coauthors and the interpersonal psychotherapy community of supervisors and practitioners. Through their interpersonal focus and basic goodness, they have increased my sense of belonging. I hope this book can provide you with tools to give a similar experience to your clients.

—Scott Fairhurst

To my family and especially to my coauthors, interpersonal psychotherapy colleagues, and the entire interpersonal psychotherapy community who have taught me so much about how to be compassionate and supportive toward others. And to Russ Noyes, who undoubtedly would have read this book, praised it, and then noted that it still could be shortened a bit.

—Scott Stuart

Contents

Series Preface

Tony Rousmaniere and Alexandre Vaz

We are pleased to introduce the Essentials of Deliberate Practice series of training books. We are developing this book series to address a specific need that we see in many psychology training programs. The issue can be illustrated by the training experiences of Mary, a hypothetical second-year graduate school trainee. Mary has learned a lot about mental health theory, research, and psychotherapy techniques. Mary is a dedicated student; she has read dozens of textbooks, written excellent papers about psychotherapy, and receives near-perfect scores on her course exams. However, when Mary sits with her clients at her practicum site, she often has trouble performing the therapy skills that she can write and talk about so clearly. Furthermore, Mary has noticed herself getting anxious when her clients express strong reactions, such as hopelessness, skepticism about therapy, or becoming very emotional. Sometimes this anxiety is strong enough to make Mary freeze at key moments, limiting her ability to help those clients.

During her weekly individual and group supervision, Mary's supervisor gives her advice informed by empirically supported therapies and common factor methods. The supervisor often supplements that advice by leading Mary through role-plays, recommending additional reading, or providing examples from her own work with clients. Mary, a dedicated supervisee who shares tapes of her sessions with her supervisor, is open about her challenges, carefully writes down her supervisor's advice, and reads the suggested readings. However, when Mary sits back down with her clients, she often finds that her new knowledge seems to have flown out of her head, and she is unable to enact her supervisor's advice. Mary finds this problem to be particularly acute with the clients who are emotionally evocative.

Mary's supervisor, who has received formal training in supervision, uses supervisory best practices, including the use of video to review supervisees' work. She would rate Mary's overall competence level as consistent with expectations for a trainee at Mary's developmental level. But even though Mary's overall progress is positive, she experiences some recurring problems in her work. This is true even though the supervisor is confident that she and Mary have identified the changes that Mary should make in her work.

The problem with which Mary and her supervisor are wrestling—the disconnect between her knowledge about psychotherapy and her ability to reliably perform psychotherapy—is the focus of this book series. We started this series because most therapists experience this disconnect, to one degree or another, whether they are beginning trainees or highly experienced clinicians. In truth, we are all Mary.

To address this problem, we are focusing this series on the use of deliberate practice, a method of training specifically designed for improving reliable performance of complex skills in challenging work environments (Rousmaniere, 2016, 2019; Rousmaniere et al., 2017). Deliberate practice entails experiential, repeated training with a particular skill until it becomes automatic. In the context of psychotherapy, this involves two trainees role-playing as a client and a therapist, switching roles every so often, under the guidance of a supervisor. The trainee playing the therapist reacts to client statements, ranging in difficulty from beginner to intermediate to advanced, with improvised responses that reflect fundamental therapeutic skills.

To create these books, we approached leading trainers and researchers of major therapy models with these simple instructions: Identify essential skills for your therapy model where trainees often experience a disconnect between cognitive knowledge and performance ability—in other words, skills that trainees could write a good paper about but often have challenges performing, especially with challenging clients. We then collaborated with the authors to create deliberate practice exercises specifically designed to improve reliable performance of these skills and overall responsive treatment (Hatcher, 2015; Stiles et al., 1998; Stiles & Horvath, 2017). Finally, we rigorously tested these exercises with trainees and trainers at multiple sites around the world and refined them based on extensive feedback.

Each book in this series focuses on a specific therapy model, but readers will notice that most exercises in these books touch on common factor variables and facilitative interpersonal skills that researchers have identified as having the most impact on client outcome, such as empathy, verbal fluency, emotional expression, persuasiveness, and problem focus (e.g., Anderson et al., 2009; Norcross et al., 2019). Thus, the exercises in every book should help with a broad range of clients. Despite the specific theoretical model(s) from which therapists work, most therapists place a strong emphasis on pantheoretical elements of the therapeutic relationship, many of which have robust empirical support as correlates or mechanisms of client improvement (e.g., Norcross et al., 2019). We also recognize that therapy models have already-established training programs with rich histories, so we present deliberate practice not as a replacement but as an adaptable, transtheoretical training method that can be integrated into these existing programs to improve skill retention and help ensure basic competency.

About This Book

The 12th book in the Essentials of Deliberate Practice series is on interpersonal psychotherapy (IPT), a time-limited psychotherapy that focuses on interpersonal issues that are understood to be a factor in the genesis and maintenance of psychological distress. The targets of IPT are symptom resolution, improved interpersonal functioning, and increased social support (Stuart & Robertson, 2012). IPT is best implemented with clients who are presenting with an interpersonal nature of distress. It is a unique relational therapeutic method, and many trainees find that a multifaceted approach to learning is required to achieve IPT competence. Competency in the clinical area requires mastery of knowledge, skills, and attitudes. We have received feedback from clinicians indicating that reading on the IPT theory, practicing IPT skills, and receiving constructive feedback from peers or supervisors is incredibly helpful. Lastly, understanding the mechanism of change within IPT will help clinicians find an appropriate attitude and relational stance with this approach. Practicing IPT skills, with ongoing feedback, will allow the clinician to calibrate their practice and help them ultimately to integrate their knowledge and skills into deeper IPT clinical practice.

In this book, we adopt deliberate practice methods to support experiential—"learning by doing"—training opportunities. The methods and stimuli described in this volume can facilitate practice of a range of important IPT skills. In addition, it supports fine-tuning the "how" of intervention delivery, including in a flexible manner across diverse clinical scenarios. Importantly, this book is not intended to replace core coursework and exposure to foundational IPT theory and principles of practice. Rather, it is intended to augment other common training components.

Thank you for including us in your journey toward psychotherapy expertise. Now let's get to practice!

Acknowledgments

We would like to acknowledge Rodney Goodyear for his significant contribution to starting and organizing this book series. We are grateful to Susan Reynolds, David Becker, Elizabeth Budd, Joe Albrecht, and Emily Ekle at American Psychological Association (APA) Books for providing expert guidance and insightful editing that has significantly improved the quality and accessibility of this book. We would also like to acknowledge the International Deliberate Practice Society and its members for their many contributions and support for our work.

The exercises in this book series have undergone extensive testing at training programs around the world. Over 130 testers (trainees, therapists, and supervisors) from 16 countries contributed to testing the exercises. For everyone who volunteered to "test run" this work and provided critically important feedback throughout the method refinement and writing process, we cannot thank you enough.

Olga Belik, Jessica M. Schultz, Scott Fairhurst, and Scott Stuart offer our joint gratitude to Kirsten Ramirez, whose organizational and administrative assistance within the IPT Institute has been invaluable in helping to produce this book and in supporting all of our interpersonal psychotherapy (IPT) training. We deeply appreciate the opportunity to work together with our wise editors—Alexandre Vaz and Tony Rousmaniere. We thank you for your guidance and patience!

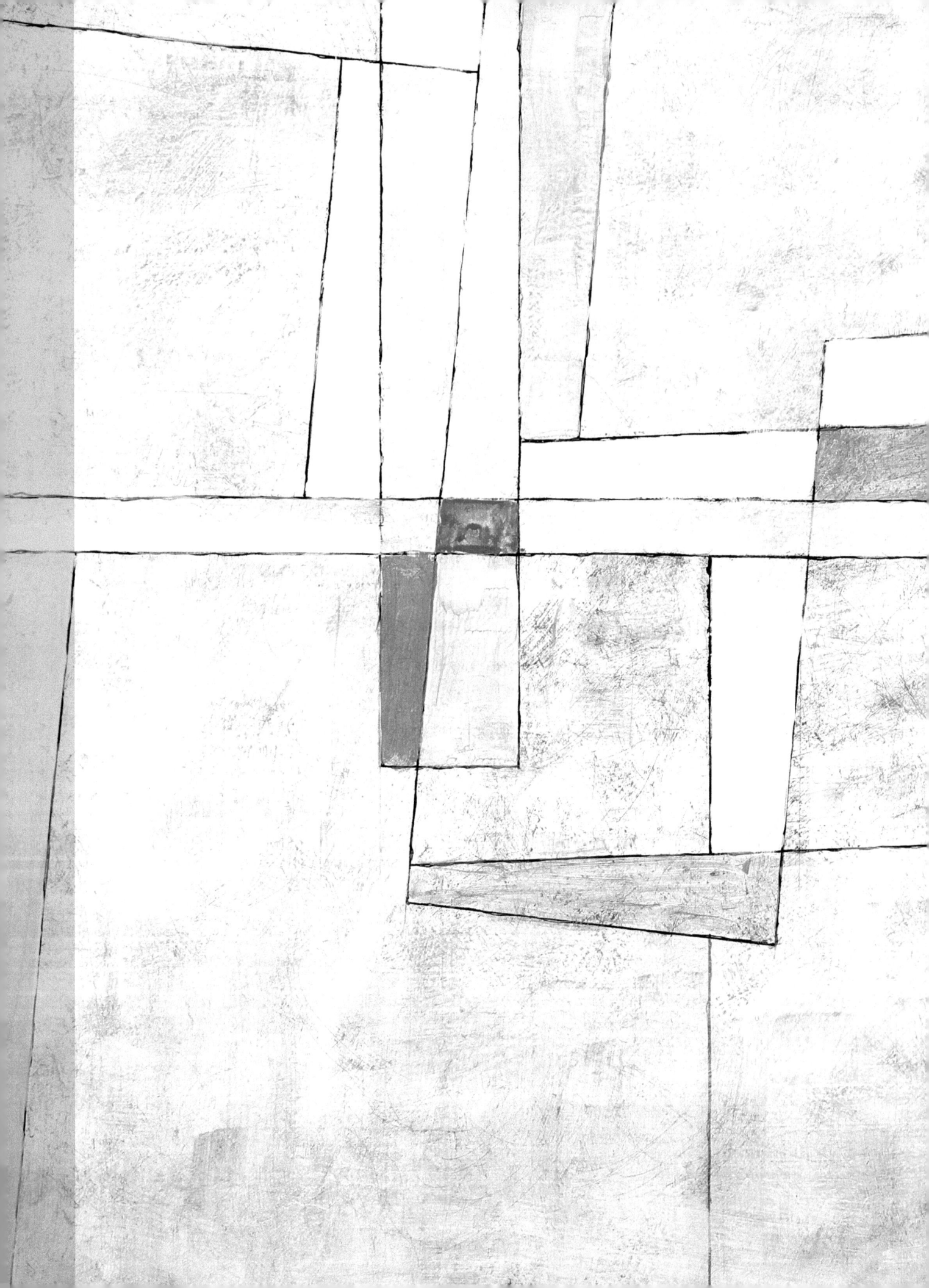

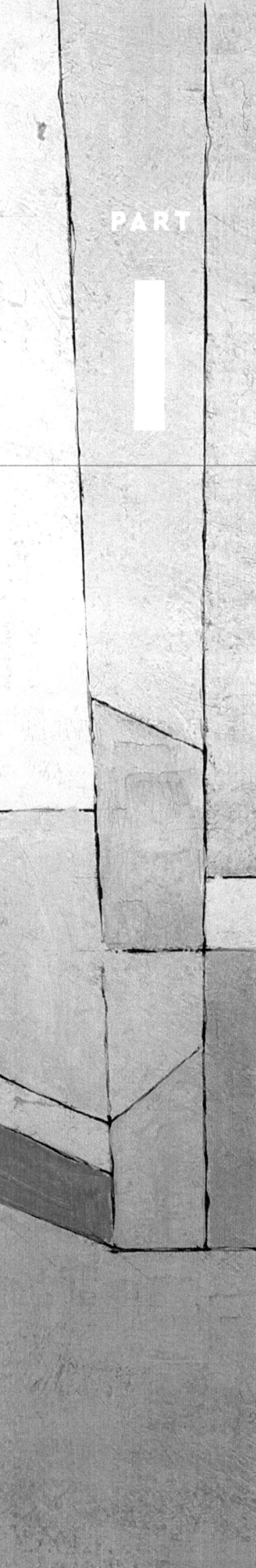

Overview and Instructions

In Part I, we provide an overview of deliberate practice, including how it can be integrated into clinical training programs for deliberate practice in interpersonal psychotherapy, and instructions for performing the deliberate practice exercises in Part II. **We encourage both trainers and trainees to read both Chapters 1 and 2 before performing the deliberate practice exercises for the first time.**

Chapter 1 provides a foundation for the rest of the book by introducing important concepts related to deliberate practice and its role in psychotherapy training more broadly and interpersonal psychotherapy training more specifically. We also individually review the 10 skills from these exercises.

Chapter 2 lays out the basic, most essential instructions for performing the interpersonal psychotherapy deliberate practice exercises in Part II. They are designed to be quick and simple and provide you with just enough information to get started without being overwhelmed by too much information. Chapter 3 in Part III provides more in-depth guidance, which we encourage you to read once you are comfortable with the basic instructions in Chapter 2.

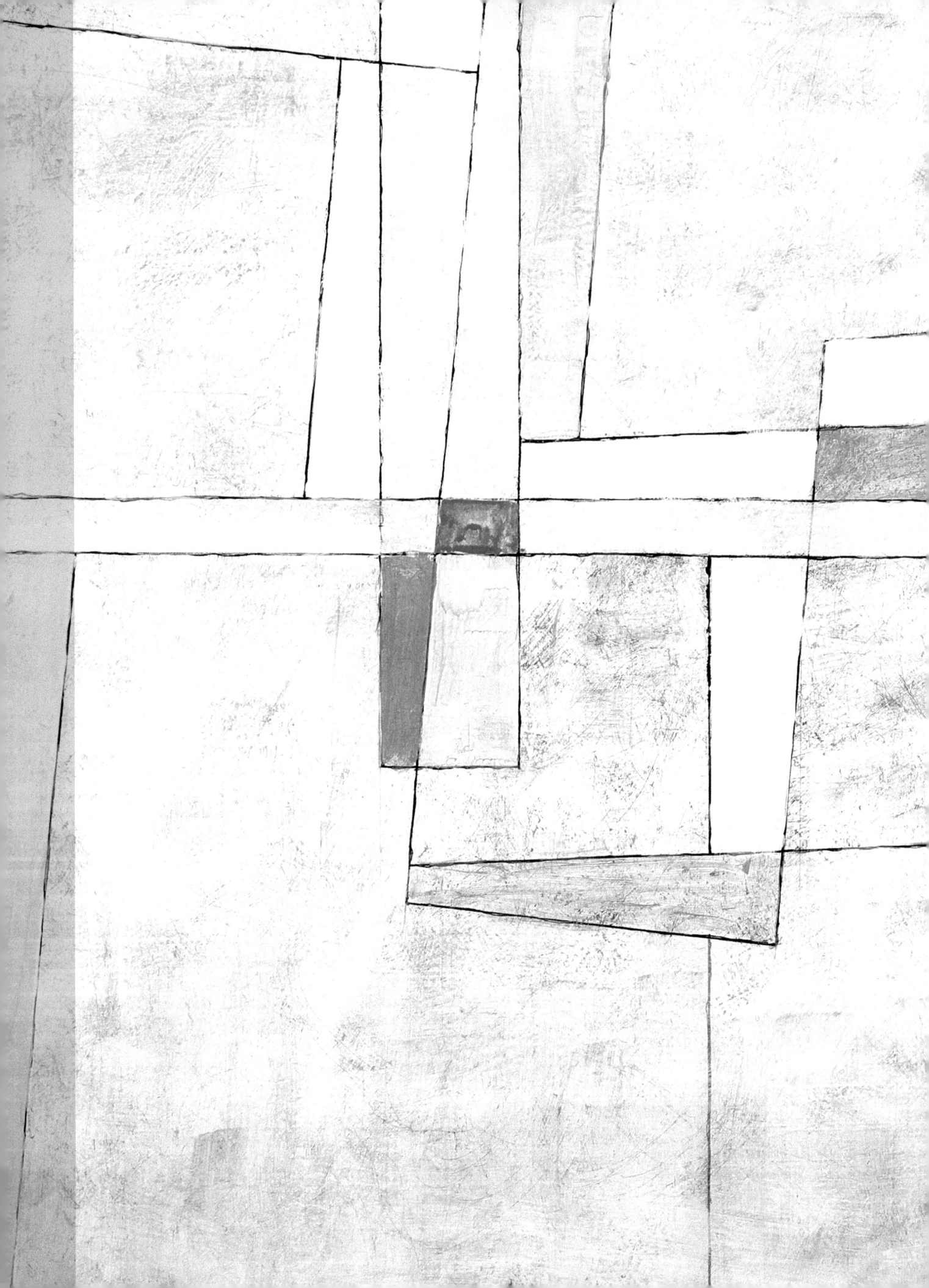

Introduction and Overview of Deliberate Practice and Interpersonal Psychotherapy

This book is designed to facilitate the acquisition of the basic skills of interpersonal psychotherapy (IPT). IPT is situated within a rich tradition of psychotherapy training, with a strong emphasis on experiential learning. Deliberate practice is a methodology used by professionals from across many fields that is being applied in psychotherapy training and can be used as an innovative way to enhance the experiential training process for IPT. Through continual practice, fundamental IPT skills eventually become natural. If practice is done effectively, this will provide the trainee the opportunity to draw on the skill automatically when presented with an appropriate moment in a real therapy session.

The fundamental basis for IPT is the *relational frame*. This simple concept means that the client's experience of distress affects the people around them and that people in the client's social support network influence the client's experience of distress. Take, for instance, the experience of distress that might be labeled, in diagnostic nomenclature, depression. The client's distress manifests itself interpersonally, cognitively, behaviorally, and spiritually as withdrawal, low self-esteem, lack of motivation, irritability, hopelessness, and even suicidality, and this profoundly affects those around them. Others may begin to feel distressed as well if the client expresses anger at them, and their distress may increase even more if others feel helpless to understand and stop the individual's thoughts of suicide, not to mention their responses to an actual suicide attempt.

Similarly, the client's friends, family, and community have a profound impact on the client's experience of distress. Consistent, supportive care and understanding from others will likely help alleviate the client's distress. Feeling "understood" and "felt by others" will decrease their distress even further.

Even cultural values, expressed by individuals within the client's community, will influence the client's distress. A cultural taboo against mental health, seeking treatment, or "airing dirty laundry" will exacerbate distress. A cultural norm—expressed in relationships—that the client should "buck up and deal with it" will also increase the client's sense of isolation and distress.

https://doi.org/10.1037/0000426-001

Deliberate Practice in Interpersonal Psychotherapy, by O. Belik, J. M. Schultz, S. Fairhurst, S. Stuart, A. Vaz, and T. Rousmaniere

The basic principle of IPT is that as humans, we are relational. Relationships matter to us; we are embedded in relationships and community. We affect others, and other people affect us. Our interpersonal communications, cognitions, behaviors, and even our spirituality take place within a relational frame. We are always interacting with others. And those interactions can help or hinder us. When we have a positive relational connection, we feel seen, understood, and have more emotional and cognitive energy to face the world and address potential challenges.

Conversely, much of our distress comes from difficulties within relationships. Those that end through death or disruption, that are in conflict, or in which we struggle to adapt and change increase our distress and isolation. The way in which we ask for help in those crises makes a difference too, as does our inability or reluctance to ask for help. So does the response from others: Reactions of understanding and compassion will be helpful, while lack of support, rejection, or judgment will make the distress worse.

Asking for help and support in an effective way is a function of communication. Communication is a learned skill and can be taught to clients. It can be taught by modeling, reinforcing, and practicing both in session using role-playing as well as out of session with "practice" in which the client engages in asking for help (or practices other communication skills learned during the session) with others in their Interpersonal Circle.

Because communication is such a critical mediator of change in IPT, the IPT clinician must learn to communicate well. Modeling good communication skills, not to mention teaching them, requires expertise on the part of the clinician. Hence, the deliberate practice approach to mastering language and communication skills is directly applicable for IPT clinicians. In this book, we have taken the opportunity both to teach clinicians to communicate more effectively in therapy and, on a metalevel, to teach clinicians how to teach their clients to communicate more effectively using the same communication skills.

It is always useful, both in teaching and in clinical care, to give practical examples to illustrate key concepts. Storytelling is a critical skill in IPT because it is a way to gain a better understanding of the concept and to make an abstract concrete.

An Interpersonal Psychotherapy Case Example

About a year ago, although it could have been a decade ago, or last month, or even yesterday, a woman came to see one of us after she experienced a miscarriage. The loss was at 12 weeks; she had already told her family and friends about her pregnancy and had been excited and expectant, as she and her partner had been trying for more than 2 years to have a baby.

Consistent with her personal and spiritual experiences, she described the miscarriage as the loss of her child. She described her distress as feeling incredibly lonely and isolated, sad, inert, and hopeless. She even had some thoughts of suicide so that she could be with her child, although she made clear that her religious beliefs would keep her from acting on these thoughts. For her, the most impactful distress came from her experience of being alone in her grief; no one else understood what her loss was like, and her sense of being alone, misunderstood, and even judged by others, was devastating.

The first thing we discussed about her loss was what words she used to understand and describe it. For her, it was, without a doubt, the death of a child. A real person who was forming inside of her body, with whom she was in the most intimate relationship a person could have with another. And she was responsible for that child. Because it was growing inside of her and because her job was to protect and keep it alive, her body had failed her. And in her mind, this meant she had failed her child.

We began discussing the ways others had responded to her grief—the ways in which the people in her relational space were responding. No one, she said, understood her grief, and all her friends and family members were making her distress even worse.

Hers is a universal experience—a lack of interpersonal connection and support—that we could have heard described a decade ago, last month, or even last week. Or even a lifetime ago.

After asking her to complete her Interpersonal Inventory to gain a better understanding of her relationships and connections, we talked about how she had told others of her experience and distress. Most others, including her mother, had responded with a comment or two about how difficult her loss must have been, followed by comments such as, "At least the miscarriage was only 12 weeks—it could have been 20 or 30, and that would have been even worse." Or "You can always get pregnant again." Or "It was only a miscarriage; it's not like you lost a child." Perhaps they were trying to be of help; perhaps they were simply inept. But she—rightly so—experienced all these experiences as rejection, misunderstanding, and disconnection. And she isolated herself even more.

We discussed several interpersonal incidents in which these specific communications had happened and discovered that as soon as she received comments from others about her loss, she would withdraw in anger at being misunderstood and unsupported. Eventually the topic became taboo because those who were trying to be supportive but did not know how to do it well learned that trying to be supportive was met with rejection—it made things worse. And the cycle of isolation, anger, and silence spiraled into even more distress.

A change point in therapy started to occur initially when she felt "seen" and "understood" by her clinician. After working hard to establish a therapeutic alliance by listening well, being empathic, and grieving with the client, I remarked that others, although perhaps trying to be sympathetic, were missing her perspective, missing the mark. Rather than being helpful, the comments such as "hang in there, you'll get over this eventually" were not helpful at all to her—they were making things worse. They were causing her to withdraw, shut down, and isolate herself even more. In the midst of her isolation, she understood what she needed from other people—she wanted a different response conveying empathy and support. Helping others to understand her experience and learning how to ask for support from others directly became one of our primary tasks in therapy.

The first step in that process was to help her describe her experience of loss and her distress in therapy. Making her implicit internal narrative explicit helped the client find words describing her experience and brought clarity to her; she was able to frame it as the loss of a child so that others could better understand the impact it was having on her. We worked to help her describe the support she needed as well—the practical, emotional, and spiritual care she needed. Looking back to the Interpersonal Inventory, we talked about whom she could begin sharing her loss experience with and who would be receptive. We then practiced the conversations in session using generating options, modeling, and role-playing, focusing on what she needed and how she could ask for it directly and effectively.

With that help and her newfound motivation and confidence to ask for the support and understanding she really needed, the client first shared her experience with her partner and then moved on to discuss it with several close friends. They were, fortunately, able to respond well to her request simply to listen and understand, not to offer advice or platitudes, and to comfort her with a hug.

This clinical case had several complexities embedded in it and represents well the reality of interpersonal distress that we encounter daily in our work. As relational human beings, we need others to understand our experiences, to feel "felt" by others on a daily basis—and even more so during a crisis. We need to be supported emotionally, practically, physically, and spiritually. Support and understanding from others improved our functioning.

Overview of the Deliberate Practice Exercises

The focus of this book is a series of 10 exercises that have been thoroughly tested and modified based on feedback from IPT trainers and trainees. The first two focus on collecting baseline information about the client's relationships and general social support and are used in the initial or assessment phase of IPT. The next four are used throughout IPT; clarification in particular is foundational in IPT. The last four skills are designed to help move the client to action—to improve their communication and then to implement their newly practiced communication skills in relationships outside of therapy. Table 1.1 presents the 10 skills that are covered in these exercises.

Throughout the exercises, trainees should work in pairs under the guidance of a supervisor and role-play as a client and a therapist, switching back and forth between the two roles. (Note that "therapist" and "clinician" are used interchangeably throughout the book.) Each of the 10 skill-focused exercises consists of multiple client statements grouped by difficulty—beginner, intermediate, and advanced—that call for a specific skill. For each skill, trainees are asked to read through and absorb the description of the skill, its criteria, and some clinical examples demonstrating how to apply it. The trainee playing the client should then read the statements, which present various prompts and challenges from clients. The trainee playing the therapist should then respond in a way that demonstrates the specific skill. Trainee therapists will have the option of practicing a response using the one supplied in the exercise or improvising and supplying one of their own.

After each client statement and therapist response couplet is practiced several times, the trainee should pause to receive feedback from the supervisor. Guided by the supervisor, the trainee will be instructed to try statement–response couplets several times, working their way through the examples. In consultation with the supervisor, trainees can go through all the exercises, starting with the least challenging and then moving to the more advanced levels. The triad (supervisor–client–therapist) will have the opportunity to discuss whether exercises present too much or too little of a challenge and to adjust them depending on their assessment.

After the first 10 exercises are two comprehensive exercises, an annotated IPT transcript and improvised mock therapy sessions, that teach practitioners how to integrate all 10 skills into more expansive clinical scenarios.

TABLE 1.1. The 10 Interpersonal Psychotherapy Skills Presented in the Deliberate Practice Exercises

Beginner Skills	Intermediate Skills	Advanced Skills
1. Presenting the Interpersonal Inventory: Interpersonal Inventory I 2. Exploring interpersonal relationships: Interpersonal Inventory II 3. Clarifications	4. Interpersonal framing of distress 5. Helping the client to describe their distress and need for support 6. Reinforcement of effective communication	7. Communication analysis 8. Generating communication options 9. Mobilizing social support 10. Motivating interpersonal action

Trainees, in consultation with supervisors, can decide which skills they wish to work on and for how long. In our testing experience, we have found practice sessions should last about an hour to receive maximum benefit.

Ideally, beginning IPT therapists will both gain confidence and achieve competence through practicing these exercises. Competence is defined here as the ability to perform an IPT skill in a manner that is flexible and responsive to the client. Skills have been chosen that are considered essential to IPT and that practitioners often find challenging to implement.

The skills identified in this book are not comprehensive in the sense of representing all one needs to learn to become a competent IPT clinician. Some will present particular challenges for trainees; we have endeavored to re-create actual interactions with real clients as best we can, and the challenges are the types that occur frequently in clinical practice. We hope that the challenges will stimulate more practice and encourage therapists to seek out more formal training in IPT.

Before presenting the exercises, we would like to give a brief description of deliberate practice methodology followed by an overview of IPT to explain how we have combined them.

The Goals of This Book

The primary goal of this book is to help trainees achieve competence in core IPT skills. Of course, the expression of those skills or competencies may look somewhat different across clients or even within a session with the same client, hence the need to practice with slightly different prompts and different clinical contexts.

The IPT deliberate practice exercises are designed to help IPT therapists develop the ability to apply IPT specific skills across a range of clinical situations by providing IPT therapists with the following opportunities:

- to develop a particular skill using a style and language that is congruent with who they are,
- to use the IPT skills in response to varying client statements and effects, and
- to try out different responses and then to receive feedback about them and ways that they might be further improved.

The practice of these skills is designed to move them into procedural memory (Squire, 2004) so that IPT therapists can access them "in the moment" during therapy, even when they are tired, stressed, overwhelmed, or discouraged. And deliberate practice is designed to build confidence to use these skills in a broad range of circumstances within different clinical contexts. We also aim to help trainees discover their own personal learning style so that they can continue their professional development long after their formal training is concluded.

Who Can Benefit From This Book?

This book is designed to be used in multiple contexts, including in graduate-level courses, supervision, postgraduate training, and continuing education programs. It assumes the following:

1. The trainer/supervisor is knowledgeable about and competent in IPT.

2. The trainer/supervisor is able to provide good demonstrations and model well how to use IPT skills across a range of therapeutic situations, via role-play and/or video.

Alternatively, the trainer may have access to examples of IPT being demonstrated using videos of expert IPT therapists.

3. The trainer/supervisor is able to provide quality feedback to students about their implementation of IPT skills.

4. Trainees will have additional materials, such as books, articles, and video demonstrations, that explain the theory, research, and rationale of IPT and each particular skill. Recommended reading for each skill is provided in the sample syllabus (Appendix D).

The exercises covered in this book series were piloted in training sites from 16 countries across four continents (North America, South America, Europe, and Asia). This book is designed for trainers and trainees from different cultural backgrounds worldwide. For further guidance on how to improve multicultural deliberate practice skills, see the book *Deliberate Practice in Multicultural Therapy* (Harris et al., 2024).

This book is also designed for those who are training at all career stages, from beginning trainees, including those who have never worked with real clients, to seasoned therapists. All exercises feature guidance for assessing and adjusting the difficulty to target the needs of each individual learner precisely. The term *trainee* is used broadly, referring to anyone in the field of professional mental health who is endeavoring to acquire or improve their IPT skills.

Deliberate Practice in Psychotherapy Training

How does one become an expert in their professional field? What can we be "trained" to do, and what is simply beyond our reach due to innate or uncontrollable factors? Questions such as these touch on our fascination with expert performers and their development. A mixture of awe and admiration surround people such as Mozart, Leonardo da Vinci, or contemporary individuals such as Serena Williams, Michael Jordan, or Caitlin Clark. What accounts for their consistently superior professional results? Evidence suggests that the amount of time spent on a particular type of training is a key factor in developing expertise in virtually all domains (Ericsson & Pool, 2016). Deliberate practice is an evidence-based method that can improve performance in an effective and reliable manner.

The concept of deliberate practice has its origins in a classic study by K. Anders Ericsson and colleagues (1993). They found that the amount of time practicing a skill and the quality of the time spent doing so were key factors predicting acquisition and mastery. They identified five key activities in learning and mastering skills: (a) observing one's own work, (b) getting expert feedback, (c) setting small incremental learning goals just beyond the performer's ability, (d) engaging in repetitive behavioral rehearsal of specific skills, and (e) continuously assessing performance. Ericsson and his colleagues termed this process deliberate practice, a cyclical process that is illustrated in Figure 1.1.

Research has shown that lengthy engagement in deliberate practice is associated with expert performance across a variety of professional fields, such as medicine, sports, music, chess, computer programming, and mathematics (Ericsson et al., 2018). People may associate deliberate practice with the widely known "10,000-hour rule" popularized by Malcolm Gladwell in his 2008 book *Outliers*. Gladwell's book, however, perpetuated two common misperceptions. The first is that 10,000 is the number of hours of practice needed to attain expertise, no matter the domain. In fact, there can be considerable variability (Ericsson & Pool, 2016). The second is that engagement in 10,000 hours of work performance will lead one to become an expert. This misunderstanding holds

FIGURE 1.1. Cycle of Deliberate Practice

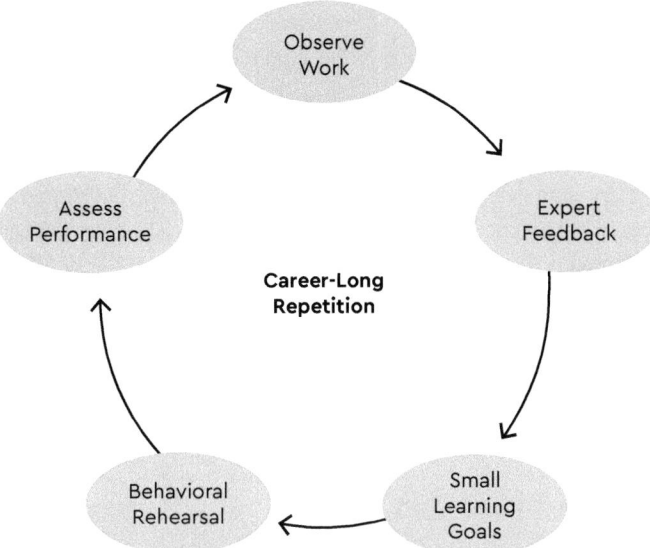

Note. From *Deliberate Practice in Emotion-Focused Therapy* (p. 7), by R. N. Goldman, A. Vaz, and T. Rousmaniere, 2021, American Psychological Association (https://doi.org/10.1037/0000227-000). Copyright 2021 by the American Psychological Association.

considerable significance for the field of psychotherapy, where hours of work experience with clients has traditionally been used as a measure of proficiency (Rousmaniere, 2016). In fact, research suggests that the amount of experience alone does not predict therapist effectiveness (Goldberg et al., 2016); it appears instead that the quality of deliberate practice is a key factor.

Psychotherapy scholars, recognizing the value of deliberate practice in other fields, have called for deliberate practice to be incorporated into training for mental health professionals (e.g., Bailey & Ogles, 2019; Hill et al., 2020; Rousmaniere et al., 2017; Taylor & Neimeyer, 2017; Tracey et al., 2015). There are, however, good reasons to question analogies made between psychotherapy and other professional fields, such as sports or music, because by comparison psychotherapy is more complex and freeform. Sports have clearly defined goals, and classical music follows a written score. In contrast, the practice and implementation of psychotherapy skills shift with the unique presentation of each client at each session. Therapists do not have the luxury of following a score.

Instead, good psychotherapy is more like improvisational jazz (Noa Kageyama, cited in Rousmaniere, 2016). In jazz improvisations, a complex mixture of group collaboration, creativity, and interaction are co-created between master musicians. Like psychotherapy, no two jazz improvisations are identical. However, improvisations are not a random collection of notes. They are grounded in a comprehensive theoretical understanding and technical proficiency that is developed through continuous deliberate practice. For example, prominent jazz instructor Jerry Coker (1990) lists 18 skill areas that students must master, each of which has multiple discrete skills including tone quality, intervals, chord arpeggios, scales, and patterns. More creative and artful improvisations are actually a reflection of repetitive skill practice and acquisition. As legendary jazz musician Miles Davis put it, "You have to play a long time to be able to play like yourself" (Cook, 2005, p. 112).

The ultimate goal of deliberate practice is to master IPT skills so that therapists can "play like themselves." In other words, the goal is to become so adept at the specific skills that the therapist can focus attention on the therapeutic relationship and over-arching goals of therapy—so adept that the therapist can be fully present and understand their clients rather than having to think about delivering certain techniques well.

Ongoing and effortful deliberate practice should not be an impediment to flexibility and creativity. Ideally, creativity should be enhanced with continued practice of the basics, just as virtuoso musicians practice the scales daily so that they can free themselves to focus on creativity and emotional expression.

Psychotherapy is an ever-shifting relationship with another real human being, and it is not and should not become formulaic. Strong IPT therapists integrate skills acquired through practice with flexibility. IPT, as noted later, also involves a way of being with the client; to be with someone therapeutically requires focus and attention.

The core IPT responses provided in subsequent exercises are meant as templates or possibilities, rather than "correct answers." Please use and apply them in a way that makes sense to you, and as you master them, be creative. We encourage flexible and improvisational play!

Simulation-Based Mastery Learning

Deliberate practice uses simulation-based mastery learning (Ericsson, 2004; McGaghie et al., 2014). The stimulus material for training presented in this book consists of "contrived social situations that mimic problems, events, or conditions that arise in professional encounters" (McGaghie et al., 2014, p. 375). A key component of this approach is that the stimuli being used in training are sufficiently similar to real-world experiences so that they provoke similar reactions. This facilitates state-dependent learning, in which clinicians acquire and practice skills in the same psychological environment where they will perform them (Fisher & Craik, 1977). Pilots, for example, train with flight simulators that present mechanical failures and dangerous weather conditions. Surgeons practice with surgical simulators that present medical complications. Training in simulations with challenging stimuli increases professionals' capacity to perform effectively under stress. For the psychotherapy training exercises in this book, the "simulators" are typical client statements that might be presented in therapy sessions and call upon the use of the particular skill.

Declarative Versus Procedural Knowledge

Declarative knowledge is that which a person can understand, write, or speak about. It often refers to factual information that can be consciously recalled through memory and is often acquired relatively quickly. In contrast, procedural learning is implicit in memory and "usually requires repetition of an activity, and associated learning is demonstrated through improved task performance" (Koziol & Budding, 2012, p. 2694). Procedural knowledge is that which a person can perform, especially under stress (Squire, 2004).

There is a big difference between their declarative and procedural knowledge. An "armchair quarterback," for example, is someone who understands and talks about athletics well (or at least thinks they understand well) but would have trouble performing when being chased by a 300-pound defensive tackle. Likewise, most dance, music, or theater critics have a very keen ability to write critically about their areas but would be unable to perform.

The sweet spot for deliberate practice is the gap between declarative and procedural knowledge. In other words, effortful practice should target those skills that the learner could write a good paper about but would have trouble actually performing with a real client.

Clinicians start with declarative knowledge, learning skills theoretically and observing others perform them. Once learned intellectually, deliberate practice fosters development of procedural learning, with the aim of therapists having "automatic" access to each of the skills that they can use when necessary.

Although this book focuses on specific IPT skill acquisition and mastery, doing so requires a basic knowledge of IPT generally. What follows is an overview of IPT; we encourage readers to review the suggested readings in Appendix D and the references and to seek out additional training in IPT.

An Overview of Interpersonal Psychotherapy

IPT is based on the fundamental principle that relationships matter; that human connection matters; that being comforted, understood, and especially being held matters. And that, especially in times of crisis, we human beings reach out to others for understanding, support, and care. This principle is directly articulated in IPT by the term *relational frame*. Humans are embedded in a social network—a family, a community, a culture—and experience relational crises within that network. Relational frame means that the individual's experience of distress impacts their social network and that the people in the distressed individual's network reciprocally impact the individual's experience. Our cognitions, behaviors, and hopes all occur within that network. The relational frame means that all human experience must be understood as social phenomena in addition to being an intrapersonal experience.

In sum, human beings are embedded in a social network. All of us at some point or another experience distress within relationships, which in return will impact our mood and our functioning.

IPT was originally developed in the 1960s by Klerman, Weissman, and Paykel, who were interested in prevention of depression relapse. The first IPT manual was written in 1984 (Klerman et al., 1984) and was used as a treatment manual for the National Institute of Mental Health Treatment of Depression Collaborative Research Program (Elkin et al., 1989), a landmark psychotherapy study that compared IPT, cognitive behavior therapy (CBT; Beck et al., 1979), the antidepressant imipramine, and placebo for the treatment of major depression.

Since the publication of the original manual, IPT has expanded to become transdiagnostic in application (Stuart & Robertson, 2012). Additionally, the theoretical grounding of IPT in attachment and interpersonal theory was added by Stuart and Robertson (2012); they also shifted the conceptual frame from a medical to the biopsychosocial–cultural–spiritual model that has been used in IPT for more than 2 decades.

The Theoretical Basis of IPT

As noted, IPT is based on both attachment and interpersonal theory, which are complementary to each other. Attachment describes the general patterns of an individual's relationships, while interpersonal theory describes how those patterns play out on a microlevel in moment-to-moment communication. Conceptualization occurs at the attachment level, but many of the IPT interventions—particularly those in this book—focus on improving direct communication to help the client increase their social support and improve their interpersonal functioning. Increasing social support and improving interpersonal functioning are change factors (mediators) in IPT.

This theoretical foundation in IPT could be described in the interpersonal triad (Figure 1.2), which explains from an IPT perspective why people become distressed (Stuart & Robertson, 2012). The process begins with an acute interpersonal crisis, such as a loss, a dispute, or difficult life change (or more than one crisis in many cases). In IPT, the term *problem area* refers to one of three general types of crises that clients often experience: role transitions, interpersonal disputes, and grief and loss. These three areas, singly or in combination, capture a great many of the interpersonal crises that clients experience.

Clients respond to interpersonal crises in a particular way because of their attachment and biopsychosocial–cultural–spiritual diathesis and are in a situation in which social support (both emotional and practical) are not sufficient to overcome their crises. The impact of interpersonal distress brings about changes in mood and functioning. Changes in one's functioning often leads to seeking help through psychotherapy.

Attachment theory was first described by John Bowlby (1969). In a break from the dominant analytic thinking of the 1950s, Bowlby theorized that humans had an instinctual drive to form relationships. Our drive to form intimate bonds is literally necessary for human survival. We function well when our attachment needs are met; we become distressed when they aren't.

Attachment organizes behavior in interpersonal relationships. It forms the basis for an enduring pattern of inner experience of the self and others that leads us to seek care and support and security from others in a characteristic way. Although heavily influenced by early childhood experiences, particularly by adverse experiences such as neglect, abuse, or abandonment, Bowlby emphasized that attachment-driven behavior continues throughout the lifespan. In IPT, it is understood that early life relationships have a profound impact on attachment style but that this impact is mediated by the quality and consistency of other relationships throughout life.

Although always operating, attachment behavior is activated when we are stressed and our sense of security is threatened. Experiences of distress such as a cancer diagnosis, the death of a loved one, or the breakup of a romantic relationship all escalate our attachment needs and lead us to seek support from others. When we are distressed, our attachment needs increase, and these attachment needs drive care-seeking behavior. We seek someone to hold us and care for us. And we do that seeking well, or not so well, by communicating our distress and our need for support to others. Hence the focus in this book on techniques to improve interpersonal communication.

Our attachment models solidify over time to become relatively rigid expectations about what all relationships are like, as well as expectations about whether others will

FIGURE 1.2. The Interpersonal Triad

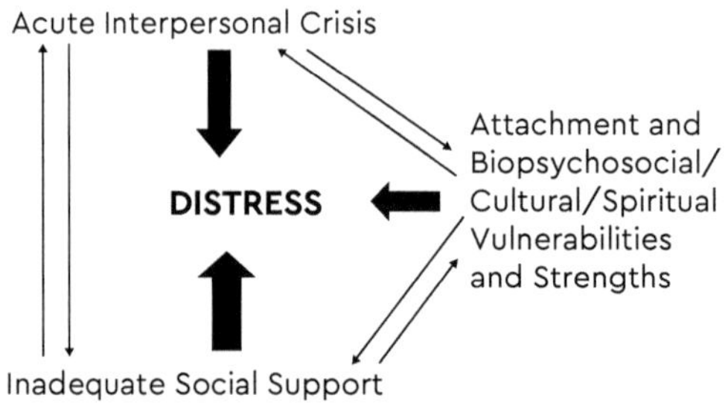

Note. Diagram is a reproduction of training material developed by the IPT Institute, LLC. Copyright IPT Institute, LLC, Scott Stuart, MD, Director. Reprinted with permission.

provide care (or not) when we need it. These internal working models of attachment guide our perceptions, emotions, and thoughts and generalize into expectations about both our current and future relationships. In other words, our cumulative relationship experiences inform our views about what our subsequent relationships will be like. And our perceptions, emotions, thoughts, and expectations eventually lead us to seek others to meet our attachment needs through interpersonal communication, which informs how we ask for help and whether we do that well or poorly.

Based on real-life experiences, individuals develop a working model of self as either being capable of caring for their own needs for the most part or as needing to rely on others for care because of their lived experience that they are incapable of caring for themselves. At the same time, based on real-life experience, they also develop a working model of others as either dependable (i.e., others are willing to provide care if asked) or as not dependable.

The IPT model of attachment (Bartholomew & Horowitz, 1991; Stuart & Robertson, 2003; Figure 1.3) is formed by the intersection of an individual's working model of self (x-axis) and their working model of others (y-axis). The intersection of the working models of self and others form the four attachment styles. People have characteristic ways of interacting with others interpersonally that are influenced by their attachment style, and those interactions are expressed in specific moment-to-moment communications, especially when they are distressed and asking for help.

There are three caveats that need to be added to the four-quadrant attachment model. First, the attachment styles are not diagnostic categories—quite the contrary. Nearly all people have characteristics of two or three styles, although often one is predominant. The best way to think about this is to envision the client occupying an area of attachment. That area may well be spread across two or more quadrants.

Second, when we become distressed, our attachment system is activated, and we tend to engage in less secure behavior. Our "area" of attachment does not change, but we move around within it. And when we are depressed, anxious, traumatized, lonely, or distressed in any of myriad ways, we tend to shift away from the secure attachment area. Distress threatens the security of our attachments.

Third, the attachment styles of other individuals we are interacting with have an influence on our care-seeking behavior as well. We engage in slightly different attachment

FIGURE 1.3. The Four Quadrant Model of Attachment in Interpersonal Psychotherapy

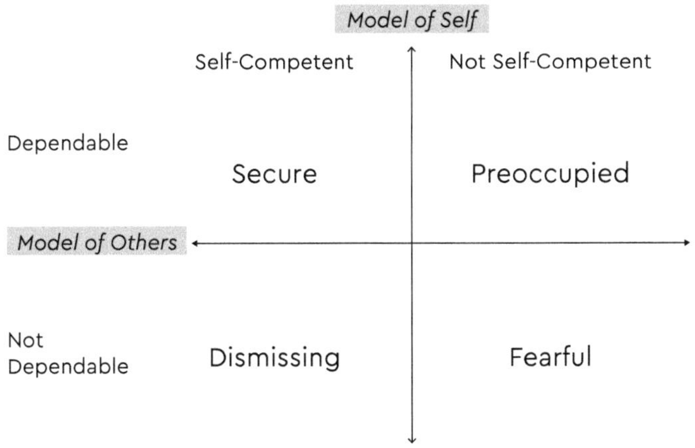

Note. Diagram is a reproduction of training material developed by the IPT Institute, LLC. Copyright IPT Institute, LLC, Scott Stuart, MD, Director. Reprinted with permission.

behaviors in different relationships. Our attachment behavior with a partner is slightly different than that with a friend, a colleague, or a parent. The other person and their attachment style always exert an influence.

As a corollary, because the other person influences a client's attachment behavior and communication, this means that we, as clinicians, have an influence on the attachment behavior we observe from clients in therapy. And this means that we need to be acutely aware of our influence and communicate in a way that models security and clarity.

The term *graciousness* describes this way of modeling and of being in IPT. Graciousness is being open, grateful, and appreciative to be in a space with a client. It is looking for the good in others, in yourself, and promoting our clients' welfare. It is coming into the therapeutic space from a secure attachment. Sometimes, on a basic level, it is simply appreciating others and expressing your gratitude by saying "thank you" and "please."

It is critical to note that communicating graciously does not preclude speaking to the truth and being direct. One can be both gracious and direct in communicating and stating needs. But it does mean being appreciative of the help and support you receive.

Graciousness is a way of being in IPT. It encompasses being present, attentive, caring, and genuine as a real human being. It includes modeling good communication so that the client can learn how to communicate well too. It is the foundational way of being—the real human relationship between yourself and your client.

You'll notice, as you go through this book, that the practical examples of statements by the clinician all include these elements of graciousness and collaboration. The IPT therapist, for example, does not direct the client to do practice or homework; instead, the IPT therapist invites the client to collaborate on homework together. The IPT therapist is quick to praise and reinforce good communication from the client. We invite you to notice these kinds of communication in the examples and to use them as a model for your own practice.

Changing a client's fundamental attachment style is incredibly difficult. The difficult task—the Sisyphean task—is that to modify their attachment style, the client would have to literally reconstruct their attachment models of self and others—not just intellectually understand them, but change them at their core. Insight isn't enough to make this change; the client would have to have many new, consistent, and real experiences of being in trusting relationships and of being self-competent over many years.

In contrast, IPT focuses on improving communication as a way of resolving here-and-now crises in the client's social network. The relational foci and points of intervention are the client's relationships with family, friends, and people in their community. IPT is focused on helping people with their current functioning—the immediate crisis—and although IPT requires an understanding of early experiences, the goal of IPT is not to change or restructure fundamental attachment styles. IPT is not designed to change the client's internal psychological structures, ego functioning, defense mechanisms, or attachment style. Instead, IPT focuses on helping the client to identify and then communicate their attachment needs more effectively and on helping them to construct a more supportive social network. Priority is given to rapid resolution of distress and improvement in interpersonal functioning.

Over a decade ago, Stuart and Robertson (2012) placed IPT within a biopsychosocial–cultural–spiritual model in recognition of the cultural and spiritual elements that are critical in understanding grief and loss, family structures, expectations about communication, and differences in social support (Schultz & Stuart, 2014). They hypothesized that interpersonal communication was directly influenced by attachment style and that communication mediated attachment and social support (Stuart & Robertson, 2012).

Combining the attachment work of Bowlby and interpersonal theorists such as Kiesler (1992; Kiesler & Watkins, 1989) and Horowitz (2004), they posited that attachment style was manifest in moment-to-moment interpersonal communications and that maladaptive interpersonal communication led to difficulties in eliciting support from others during times of distress, difficulties in resolving interpersonal conflicts, and problems in generating needed social support. The goal of IPT interventions then shifts from changing fundamental attachment style to helping clients better identify and communicate their attachment needs for support. Communication, in contrast to attachment, is a learned skill and can be modified within a short-term framework.

That is why the skills in this book are focused on communication. Improved communication is a change factor in IPT—a mediator of change. Improved communication can be learned efficiently through therapist modeling, reinforcement of good communication by the client, and of course practicing both in session and in relationships in the client's social network.

Over the past 60 years, a variety of interpersonal models have been developed based on interpersonal and communication theory (Sullivan, 1953; see also Benjamin, 1996; Horowitz, 2004; Kiesler, 1996). All of them share the concept of reciprocity or complementarity in communication: that specific interpersonal communications tend to elicit or provoke particular types of responses from others. This principle of complementarity— that the way we ask for help influences the way others are likely to respond—is a cornerstone of interpersonal theory and of IPT.

In sum, maladaptive attachment styles lead to ambiguous, ineffective, hostile, or withdrawing interpersonal communication; this elicits a negative response from others that keeps the client's attachment needs from being met. The client's verbal and nonverbal communications, especially when they are stressed, tend to elicit or provoke rejection from others. The client's distress then increases further, creating a negative spiral of worsening communication and even greater unmet needs.

It must be noted that poor interpersonal communication is frequently coupled with poor interpersonal relationships generally. In other words, it is frequently the case that it is not only that the client's communication is causing more problems but that others in their social support network are not inclined to be of help or, in some cases, are struggling with healthy communications themselves. Our clients' social networks are sometimes replete with family members who have abused them, neglected them, and who have attachment problems of their own. Thus, the focus on improving communication in IPT must be coupled with helping the client find supporters who will actually be able to understand and help. Assisting our clients' to have realistic appreciation and understanding of others' willingness and relational capability (how to "boundary" toxic relationships or protect themselves from others who will make things worse) becomes one of the aspects of the IPT work. Decreasing the space between relational expectations and reality will assist clients with the acceptance of what others can and cannot help with. When we decrease the space between expectations and reality, we let go of disappointment and can obtain the freedom to find support from other people who are not only capable but also willing to help.

Two exercises in this book are devoted to ways of doing that. The Interpersonal Inventory (Exercises 1 and 2) is designed to get a baseline assessment of the people in the client's life. Using this, the therapist can help identify who among the client's connections will be most likely to respond well to requests for support.

The primary point of intervention in IPT is therefore to assist in improving communication, which is a teachable skill. Improved communication then helps to increase needed social support. This conceptual approach directly informs the specific IPT techniques described in this book, such as the development of interpersonal incidents, communication analysis, and reinforcement of effective communication.

From Theory to Practice: The Structure, Tools, and Techniques of IPT

Individual IPT is usually delivered flexibly over approximately six to 20 sessions and can be divided into assessment/initial, middle, concluding, and maintenance phases (Figure 1.4).

The assessment/initial sessions include a general clinical assessment as well as three tasks specific to IPT. These are collaboratively constructing the Interpersonal Inventory (see Exercises 1 and 2) and the IPT Summary. The therapist should also construct an IPT formulation, which conceptualizes why the client is distressed based directly on the biopsychosocial–cultural–spiritual model.

The middle phase includes work to resolve the client's interpersonal problems within the IPT problem areas (interpersonal disputes, role transition, grief and loss). More complexity usually requires more sessions; the poorer the client's social support, the more difficult their interpersonal problems, and the less securely attached they are, the more sessions that are needed. That is why the number of sessions in IPT is flexible.

IPT is not terminated; instead, the clinician should make a shift to maintenance treatment once the client has recovered. There are several reasons for this. First, most clients we work with are at high risk of relapse. Depression is remitting and relapsing; anxiety tends to relapse; eating disorders, posttraumatic stress disorder (PTSD), substance abuse disorders, and many others relapse too. To terminate acute treatment is to leave your client at greater risk for relapse, particularly when coupled with the data that maintenance IPT does reduce relapse risk (Kupfer et al., 1992). Thus, IPT is structured to reflect the real clients with whom we work.

When concluding acute treatment, the therapist should review progress and plan for future problems, especially relapse. Sessions can be less frequent as the conclusion approaches. Maintenance IPT should be scheduled based on the client's history, severity of distress, and risk for relapse. In all cases, the goal of IPT is to conclude acute treatment when the client has recovered, and then shift to maintenance to keep them well.

FIGURE 1.4. The Structure of Interpersonal Psychotherapy (IPT)

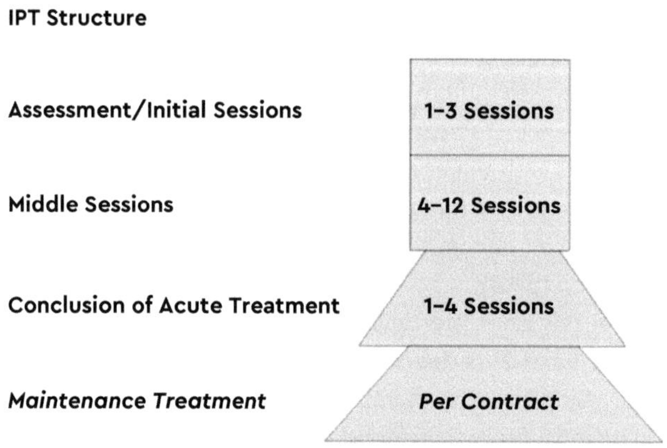

IPT Structure

Assessment/Initial Sessions	**1–3 Sessions**
Middle Sessions	**4–12 Sessions**
Conclusion of Acute Treatment	**1–4 Sessions**
Maintenance Treatment	*Per Contract*

Note. Diagram is a reproduction of training material developed by the IPT Institute, LLC. Copyright IPT Institute, LLC, Scott Stuart, MD, Director. Reprinted with permission.

Assessment/Initial Phase of IPT

The Interpersonal Inventory (Exercises 1 and 2) is a helpful assessment tool to map and evaluate the important current relationships in a client's life. It is usually conducted in Session 2 or 3. It collaboratively engages the client, helping them to understand their general social support and critical aspects of specific relationships.

The Interpersonal Inventory (or what we call at times an "Interpersonal Circle" or a "Circle") is a unique feature of IPT. Like all the IPT tools, the Interpersonal Circle (Figure 1.5) is designed to structure therapy while listening well. This is the essence of IPT: listening to the client well while using a structure that facilitates change.

The Interpersonal Circle is a simple series of concentric circles. Using a blank piece of paper, the therapist draws the two circles, then asks the client to imagine that they are in the center of the inner circle and asks them to write the names of seven to 10 (or more) people in their social support network—people relevant to the presenting problem—on the diagram. The innermost circle should include people with whom they feel intimate, the middle circle people with whom they feel close, and the outermost area those who are extended supports. The goal is to get a "big-picture" map of the client's general social support. It is helpful for the client to do the writing on the Circle because it could convey that their perspective and story is the important one.

Once names are on the Interpersonal Circle, the therapist is instructed to use open-ended questions to get a sense of the client's relationship with each person. The goal of the Interpersonal Inventory is to get a good general overview of social support, not to begin resolving specific problems. The problem-solving work will take place in the Middle Phase.

The IPT formulation and summary are two closely related tools unique to IPT. The formulation is a "formal" description of the client's current problems using technical language to denote constructs such as personality, attachment, social support, and biological risk factors. It is structured and included in the client's medical record. The summary, in contrast, is an understanding of the client's problems put in their own language. It is developed collaboratively in session and constructed with a great deal of input from the client. It is a mutually developed road map and treatment agreement for therapy.

FIGURE 1.5. The Interpersonal Circle

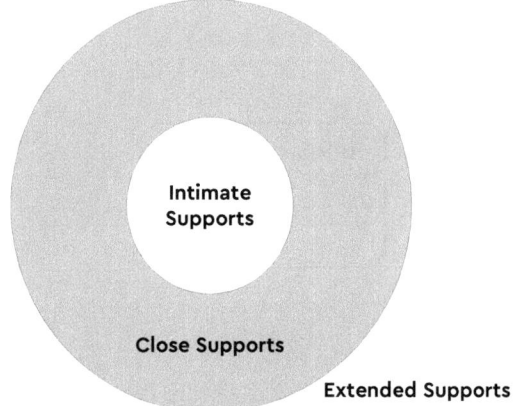

Note. "Intimate supports" are individuals who are closest to the client and who the client feels they can rely on the most. "Close supports" are individuals who are still close to the client but not as close and supportive as the intimate supports. "Extended supports" are individuals who are distant from the client and provide either limited or no support. Diagram is a reproduction of training material developed by the IPT Institute, LLC. Copyright IPT Institute, LLC, Scott Stuart, MD, Director. Reprinted with permission.

FIGURE 1.6. Interpersonal Formulation

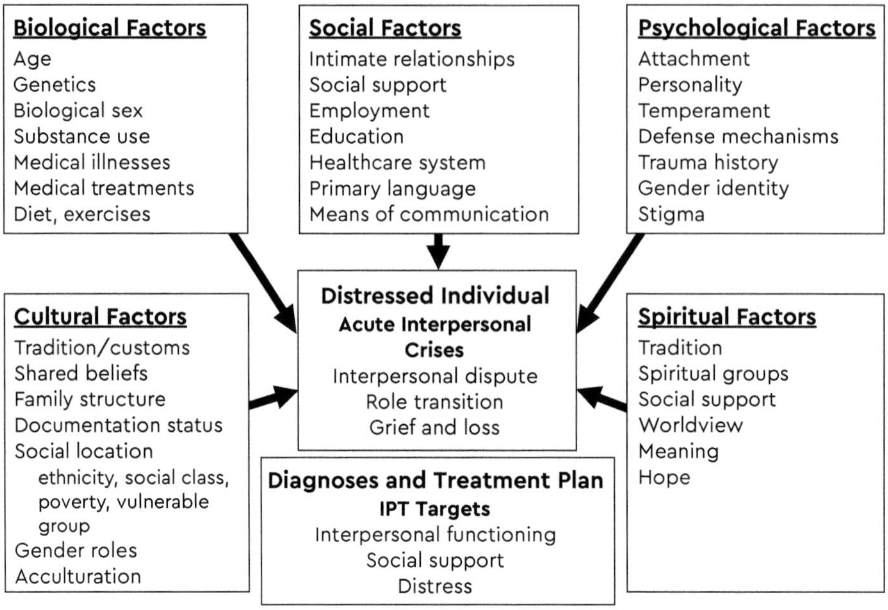

Biological Factors
Age
Genetics
Biological sex
Substance use
Medical illnesses
Medical treatments
Diet, exercises
Social Factors
Intimate relationships
Social support
Employment
Education
Healthcare system
Primary language
Means of communication
Psychological Factors
Attachment
Personality
Temperament
Defense mechanisms
Trauma history
Gender identity
Stigma
Cultural Factors
Tradition/customs
Shared beliefs
Family structure
Documentation status
Social location
ethnicity, social class, poverty, vulnerable group
Gender roles
Acculturation
Distressed Individual
Acute Interpersonal Crises
Interpersonal dispute
Role transition
Grief and loss
Spiritual Factors
Tradition
Spiritual groups
Social support
Worldview
Meaning
Hope
Diagnoses and Treatment Plan
IPT Targets
Interpersonal functioning
Social support
Distress

Note. IPT = interpersonal psychotherapy. Diagram is an adaptation of training material developed by the IPT Institute, LLC. Copyright IPT Institute, LLC, Scott Stuart, MD, Director. Adapted with permission.

Both the IPT formulation and summary are based on a biopsychosocial-cultural-spiritual model (Figure 1.6). This is reflected in the structure of the formulation, which includes information in all five of these categories. The formulation includes data from the general psychiatric and medical history, family history, and social history. It also includes information about social support from the Interpersonal Inventory. The formulation should include diagnoses and the target problem areas that will be addressed in therapy.

In contrast, the IPT summary (Figure 1.7) should contain technical language because it uses terms understandable to the client. It is the last element of the assessment,

FIGURE 1.7. The Interpersonal Summary

Reason for Distress 1
Goals
1)
2)
3)
Reason for Distress 2
Reason for Distress 3
Specific Strengths
Reason for Distress 4

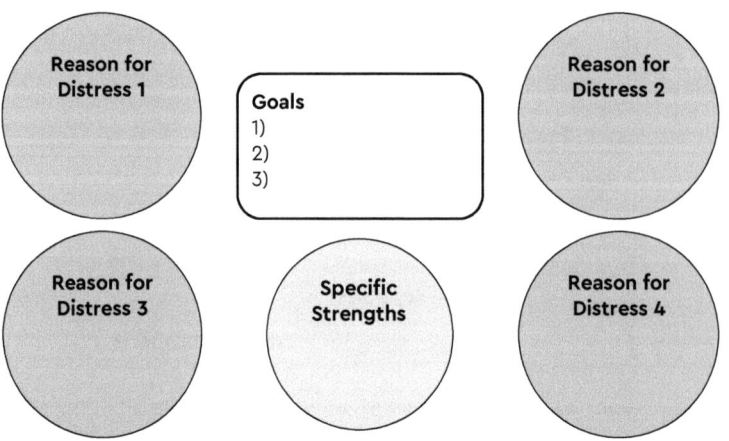

Note. Diagram is an adaptation of training material developed by the IPT Institute, LLC. Copyright IPT Institute, LLC, Scott Stuart, MD, Director. Adapted with permission.

following the general evaluation and the Interpersonal Circle. It is literally a collaboratively developed diagram written by the client in session that addresses the following questions: (a) How did their problems develop? (b) What factors are maintaining their problems? and (c) What can be done about them?

The summary is not a diagnosis; it is a collaboratively developed explanation of the client's distress that describes how their symptoms have developed and are being maintained. These "layperson" explanations should be written by the client in the four outer circles of the diagram (Reasons for Distress 1–4). The summary emphasizes the interpersonal factors involved in the origin and context of the problems and suggests the areas in which IPT will help overcome them. It is pivotal—the successful collaboration between client and therapist in developing a personally meaningful summary sets the stage for the middle phase of IPT.

The summary also contains two additional collaboratively developed elements. The first is an explicit description of the client's specific strengths. Discussing and elaborating their strengths is an important therapeutic step emphasizing their ability to overcome the crises. The summary also contains two or three collaboratively developed goals. These general goals, developed in more detail in the middle phase, are the roadmap and treatment agreement for the rest of IPT.

Middle Phase of IPT

In the middle phase, the therapist and client work together on the goals established in the summary and then work to resolve the interpersonal disputes, role transitions, grief and loss issues, or a combination of these.

Role Transitions

Change always happens as people move through life. Transitions are difficult and often require extra effort and resources even when difficulties are expected. Some reflect life-cycle changes such as adolescence, young adulthood, childbirth and becoming a parent, growing older, and changes in health generally. Others include changes in school, employment, retirement, marriage, divorce, moving, and emigration. Particular transitions are experienced very differently by individual clients, and specific and unique cultural expectations often influence them.

Successful transition requires an understanding and acceptance by the client of what they are leaving behind and what they are about to encounter. This is often accompanied by ambivalence about change, grief and loss regarding their old roles and the relationships associated with them, anxiety about their new roles, and a need for new social skills and additional social support.

The goals when working with role transitions are to assist the client in developing and articulating the complexity of their transition—their story—to relinquish an old role, to accept a new one, and to develop a sense of mastery in their new role. As the client evaluates and communicates their expectations to others, improved social support will be fostered. Because transitions occur within a social context, increased social support contributes to the adaptation to the new role.

Sequentially connecting events and symptoms allows the client to gain a realization of why and how the stressors have emerged during the transition. The primary clinical tool used to assist the client to understand their transition and describe it to others is the Life Events Timeline (Figure 1.8).

To construct a timeline, the clinician, near the beginning of the middle phase, draws a line with an arrow pointing to the right and a vertical line in the middle signifying the

FIGURE 1.8. Interpersonal Psychotherapy Life Events Timeline

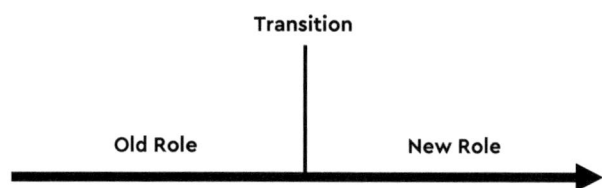

Note. Diagram is a reproduction of training material developed by the IPT Institute, LLC. Copyright IPT Institute, LLC, Scott Stuart, MD, Director. Reprinted with permission.

transition. One can visualize the old role to the left and the new role to the right. The paper is then handed to the client with instructions to mark points of relevance to their transition on the timeline.

The timeline is designed to elicit in a structured way the client's story about the events leading up to the point of transition, their current situation, and their hope for the life beyond the transition. Asking the client to complete open-ended statements about the transition greatly assists them to create a coherent story with a beginning, middle, and end. Asking open-ended questions such as "Where does the arrow go for you?" and "What do you aspire to in the future?" are extremely helpful to address forward movement—the arrow on the right of the timeline—and the inevitability of continued change. For many clients, it is helpful to start discussing where this current transition might lead them in the future and while the discussion provides them with a sense of hope as they move forward in their transition. During the discussion, which may take many sessions, the goal is to assist the client to understand and appreciate the complexity of their transition, address and resolve ambivalence about the change, and create a coherent and meaningful story that they can share with others to facilitate understanding and elicit the support and care they need to weather the transition well. Specifically, asking questions such as "What part of your story that we discussed today/ so far do you think might be helpful for someone in your life to know?" could assist others to understand the client better and elicit support.

Interpersonal Disputes

Interpersonal conflicts arise when two or more people are not communicating well and have expectations of each other that are not fulfilled. Interpersonal conflict and unmet needs lead to acute distress.

The three treatment goals associated with disputes are (a) to elaborate and understand the dispute, (b) to improve communication skills to resolve it, and (c) to broaden social support generally. At the core is work to improve the client's ability to understand and describe their needs. As people on their Interpersonal Circle who are likely to respond well are identified, the client and clinician can work on expressing and communicating their needs for support in a way that can be better understood and responded to by others.

Several IPT techniques are often used with interpersonal disputes. Connecting the dispute to affect is imperative because it facilitates change. Communication analysis followed by generating communication options helps to unveil the status of the relationship and to start setting realistic expectations about it. Evaluating expectations is important; anger and disappointment stem from expectations that are not realistic and are not explicitly stated. Assisting the client to see, accept, and appreciate others for what and how they are able and willing to support them becomes an aspect of the interpersonal disputes work that helps to close the gap between expectations and reality. Lastly, when communications do not go well, emotions arise. It might be helpful in some cases to assist clients with additional understanding and management of their emotional states so that their communications are delivered in a clear, direct, and helpful way.

Grief and Loss

Loss can lead to feelings of emptiness and isolation, often occurring in waves or "pangs of grief" and may sometimes even include thoughts of death related to the loss. The circumstances that lead to the loss can include illness, accidents, addiction, abuse, divorce, and loss of physical health, as well as anticipation of any of these. Complicating the process, grief can also be cumulative; interpersonal stress related to even seemingly minor losses, such as the transfer of a friend in the workplace, is more likely to trigger depression in people who have experienced parental loss in their childhood.

Within IPT, there is an understanding that each person's experience of grief and loss is unique. The first therapeutic step in coping better with loss is for the clinician to listen and appreciate/understand in a way that is supportive to the client and the loss that the client sustained. Some clients experience complicated, often heart-wrenching grief, and the empathy-driven experience of being and feeling understood, as well as a supportive attachment to the therapist at this vulnerable time, begins the healing process.

The clinician's second goal is to help the client to describe the loss experience, first to the therapist and then to others. During this step, the clinician can be directive with clarifying questions such as "What was your reaction when you first found out about the loss?" or "What kind of support do you hope for from others?" Clarification and helping the client to describe their distress and need for support are two specific skills that can be brought to bear. Description of the experience in therapy then becomes a bridge toward the third goal of assisting the client to connect with others—that is, mobilizing social support. This moves toward reducing isolation and meeting the client's social and attachment needs. Finally, the clinician works toward helping the client increase general social support with new or modified relationships, increasing a sense of meaning and purpose.

Conclusion and Maintenance Treatment With IPT

As noted earlier, acute treatment with IPT comes to a conclusion, not a termination. In IPT, provision is specifically made for maintenance appointments. Both clinical experience and empirical evidence consistently demonstrate that a continuing therapeutic relationship is beneficial for most clients (E. Frank et al., 1990, 2007). Because of this, the therapist is obligated to discuss maintenance treatment with all clients.

IPT can be conceptualized as a "family practice" model of care, in which short-term treatment for an acute problem is provided until it is resolved, and then maintenance treatment is provided as needed to keep the client well. The treatment is ongoing: The client is welcome to return should another acute problem arise and is encouraged to return for periodic health maintenance.

Maintenance IPT is designed to enhance the gains made in the acute phase. Clinicians should work collaboratively with clients to create a maintenance treatment plan guided by client history and context (E. Frank et al., 2007; Stuart & Robertson, 2012). Dosing of maintenance IPT might range from monthly for a client at high risk of relapse to every 6 months for one with a single episode of mild depression. In either case, it is critical that the clinician and client have a clear, collaborative agreement about maintenance sessions.

Although the maintenance phase is less intensive than acute treatment, it is not less focused. Maintenance treatment with a clear focus on interpersonal issues is significantly more effective (E. Frank et al., 1991). The acute phase is characterized by active work to improve interpersonal functioning and social support to resolve distress; the maintenance phase is refinement of the newly developed interpersonal skillset to prevent the return of distress (Stuart & Robertson, 2012).

IPT Techniques

In IPT, a good therapeutic alliance is the necessary foundation on which all techniques are built. Genuineness, graciousness, warmth, empathy, and unconditional positive regard (J. D. Frank, 1971; Rogers, 1957), although not sufficient for change in IPT, are all necessary (Stuart & Robertson, 2003, 2012). The primary goal of the IPT practitioner should be to understand the client and provide them with a sense of being understood.

Although several techniques are specific to IPT, it is the focus on current interpersonal relationships which unifies them. Many specific IPT techniques—particularly the ones covered in this book—are designed to improve the client's communication. Primary goals in IPT are to determine how the client is asking for help and support in maladaptive ways, to help them recognize that they are doing so, and to help them implement new and more effective communication. Helping the client to communicate more directly, clearly, and graciously, makes it more likely that their interpersonal problems will be resolved and social support will be more effectively engaged.

Communication analysis is one of the techniques used to help the client communicate more clearly about the help and support they want from significant others and to convey this more effectively. The first step in communication analysis is the elicitation of important interpersonal incidents (Stuart & Robertson, 2003, 2012). Interpersonal incidents are descriptions by the client of specific interactions with another person. To identify patterns of disputes with a partner, for example, the therapist can ask the client to "describe the last time you and your partner got into a fight" or to "describe one of the big conflicts you had with your partner." The therapist should direct the client to describe the communication in detail, re-creating the dialogue as accurately as possible. The client should be directed to describe their affective reactions and both verbal and nonverbal responses, and to describe observations of their partner's nonverbal behavior. The purpose of eliciting interpersonal incidents is to discover patterns—that is, to determine what is not going well with the client's communication so that steps can be taken to improve it (Stuart & Robertson, 2012).

The next step is to examine the consequences of the ineffective communication. The therapist can link this to the client's affect, and particularly to his sense of feeling misunderstood and alone. This provides the client with insight into the communication as well as motivation to change it.

Once maladaptive communication patterns are identified, the interactive process of giving feedback to the client begins. The client is encouraged to understand the dispute as a problem that can be improved with more direct communication. The client and therapist can then begin to develop possible solutions using techniques such as brainstorming and problem-solving.

Practice comes next with an emphasis on role-playing and assigning practicing the skills learned during the session/homework to engage social support. Role-playing can be used to help the client practice the interpersonal skills they have developed in session; practicing outside of the session provides the opportunity to master these interpersonal skills with people in their life and to gain self-efficacy.

IPT Clinical Applications

The application of IPT is best determined by the individual's unique problems, distress, and social context. Although research in IPT is specific to particular diagnoses or populations, restricting its use to these limits both its use and its dissemination. IPT is best thought of as a transdiagnostic approach for interpersonal problems (Stuart, 2019; Stuart & Robertson, 2003, 2012) which may be associated with a variety of diagnoses.

With respect to specific disorders, IPT has been empirically validated for affective disorders, anxiety disorders, eating disorders, and PTSD. Meta-analyses strongly support the effectiveness of IPT for depression with moderate to large effect sizes comparable to other established psychotherapies (Barth et al., 2013; Cuijpers et al., 2011, 2016, 2020, 2021). An IPT-specific meta-analysis from 2016 found it to be as effective as pharmacotherapy alone for treating depression (Cuijpers et al., 2016).

IPT is also validated for anxiety disorders. Meta-analyses of trials of IPT for anxiety disorders found large effects for IPT compared with control conditions and that IPT was equivalent to CBT (Bright et al., 2020; Cuijpers et al., 2016). IPT for anxiety is well tolerated and has low levels of attrition (Markowitz et al., 2014); meta-analytic evidence suggests the 16.1% dropout rate for IPT for anxiety disorders is significantly lower than other psychotherapies, including CBT (Linardon et al., 2019).

IPT has been validated in individual and group formats with bulimia nervosa, binge eating disorder, and anorexia nervosa (Fairburn et al., 2003). Results from a large meta-analysis showed that IPT had significant effects on all eating disorders, although the effect sizes were noted to likely be smaller than that of CBT in acute phases of treatment (Cuijpers et al., 2016). A comprehensive literature review concluded that there were no significant differences between IPT and CBT in treating anorexia (Miniati et al., 2018). Although CBT sometimes had faster gains, IPT had an equivalent improvement at follow-up. The authors concluded that IPT is a reasonable, cost-effective alternative to CBT for treating eating disorders transdiagnostically.

A meta-analysis of 10 clinical trials of IPT consisting of 755 patients with PTSD symptoms concluded that IPT had an overall effect size of 0.44 and was clearly superior to passive controls such as waitlists (Althobaiti et al., 2020). IPT appears to be as effective as other active treatments, but there are not yet enough comparative studies to draw firm conclusions. However, IPT certainly holds promise as a more tolerable and acceptable treatment for PTSD than exposure-based treatments and may be particularly effective for sexual trauma.

IPT has been used effectively with geriatric patients (Reynolds et al., 1992, 1999, 2010), adolescents (Mychailyszyn & Elson, 2018; Pu et al., 2017; Zhou et al., 2015, 2020), and perinatal women (Bright et al., 2020; O'Hara et al., 2000; Sockol, 2018; Sockol et al., 2011). It is also effective in groups (Johnson et al., 2019; Mennen et al., 2021; Mulcahy et al., 2010; Pessagno, 2013; Reay et al., 2012) and with couples (Brandon et al., 2012). IPT has been found to be effective in international settings across many cultures as well (Bass et al., 2006; Bolton et al., 2003; Cuijpers et al., 2018; Verdeli et al., 2008).

IPT Skills in Deliberate Practice

There are 10 specific IPT skills covered in this textbook. The first two exercises in the beginner section cover the Interpersonal Inventory; as noted previously, the inventory is a critical and unique tool in IPT designed to understand the client's social support network. That requires starting the exercise well by enlisting the client's cooperation

(Exercise 1) as well as getting more detailed information about each of the relationships the client lists on the inventory (Exercise 2). This provides an overview of the nature of their interpersonal support, including the quality of each specific relationship.

"Clarifications" (Exercise 3) is another skill covered in the beginner section. Clarification is used throughout IPT, both in information gathering and in exploring options for change; in addition to being a helpful tool for information gathering, it is also a way to model good communication for the client.

The intermediate section includes three intermediate level skills. The first, "Interpersonal Framing of Distress" (Exercise 4), is important because it provides a framework for both the therapist and client to understand the client's distress as arising from, and influenced by, their interpersonal relationships. Setting this framework then leads to clear goals in therapy and to work to improve interpersonal functioning and to increase social support.

Once there is a clear, collaboratively developed understanding of the client's distress, the therapist can work on helping the client to describe it, first in therapy and then to others. Describing why the client is distressed and what their experience is like is immensely helpful in generating attachment support. Once others understand better, they are more likely to respond to the client's need for help. "Helping the Client to Describe Their Distress and Need for Support" (Exercise 5) is a skill the therapist can use to accomplish that.

The last skill in the intermediate section is "Reinforcement of Effective Communication" (Exercise 6). In addition to modeling good communication, the therapist can provide direct feedback to the client in session to help them improve their communication skills. As with any behavioral change—in this case, change in communication—the best strategy is to reinforce positive change. Noticing good communication when it occurs and then reinforcing it positively is an effective way to do this.

The advanced section builds on these communication skills and begins to move them toward implementation in the client's relationships with family, friends, and people in their community. To improve communication in those relationships, examples of communication must be collected and analyzed. "Communication Analysis" (Exercise 7) is designed to do this in several steps. First, examples of specific communication (interpersonal incidents) are collected as data points for understanding what is not going well in the client's communication with others. These specific incidents collected early in therapy usually focus on interactions in which the client asked for support but did not get their needs met. In IPT, based on the relational frame conceptualization, it is always an understanding that the communication occurs within a system; it is never the "fault" of one person or another, but rather the interactive communication within a system. Those communications should also clarify the emotional experience of the client (Step 2) and the emotions they were trying to communicate to understand the interaction more fully.

It is worth noting here that the same technique of collecting and analyzing interpersonal incidents can and should be used later in therapy to highlight examples of communication which did go well and those in which the client's needs did get met. This allows the therapist to praise the client's effective and specific communication in a meaningful way and to provide positive reinforcement for it, making it even more likely that they will continue to communicate well.

Once samples are collected and examined, the third step in communication analysis is to help the client describe what they were hoping to get from the specific communication in which they were asking for help but did not get it. The therapist should guide the discussion here; although the client has very legitimate needs for support, the fact that their needs were frustrated leads to the likely conclusion that the communication within the relational system was not going well. If so, then the client can do something about it: They can practice more effective communication in session and then implement that communication with their significant other once again (Step 4).

Once it is clear to the client that their communication has not been effective, the next step is to work with them to brainstorm and develop other communication options. The appropriately titled "Generating Communication Options" (Exercise 8) is designed to do that and to help the client practice different ways of communicating in session. Communicating their experiences to others by "Mobilizing Social Support" (Exercise 9) follows, and the likelihood of implementing these new ways of communication increases using the skill of "Motivating Interpersonal Action" (Exercise 10).

The Role of Deliberate Practice in IPT Training

Deliberate practice fits well with the IPT approach to therapy, which emphasizes improving communication. On a metalevel, the skills you learn and master from these exercises should mirror those you teach your clients. Communication is a learned skill: Modeling it well, reinforcing good communication when it occurs, and practicing it within session and in real relationships will improve that skill. And that, in a nutshell, is what you personally will be doing in these exercises to improve your communication with your clients.

The earlier overview of IPT is just that—an overview. We strongly recommend engaging in more reading about IPT, particularly the theory and structure of IPT. Excellent textbooks include *Interpersonal Psychotherapy: A Clinician's Guide* (Stuart, 2019; Stuart & Robertson, 2003, 2012), which is designed specifically for clinical use, and *Interpersonal Psychotherapy for Adolescents: A Clinician's Guide* (McAlpine & Hillin, 2021), for those working with children and teens. Introductory training, advanced training, and supervision in IPT are available through the IPT Institute (https://iptinstitute.com), as are opportunities to join the community of IPT clinicians in monthly Case Conferences and mentorship groups for IPT supervisors and trainers.

Overview of the Book's Structure

This book is organized into three parts. Part I contains this chapter and Chapter 2, which provides basic instructions on how to perform these exercises. Further guidelines for getting the most about deliberate practice are provided in Chapter 3, and additional instructions for monitoring and adjusting the difficulty of the exercises are provided in Appendix A. **Do not skip the instructions in Chapter 2, and be sure to read the additional guidelines and instructions in Chapter 3 and Appendix A once you are comfortable with the basic instructions.**

Part II contains the 10 skill-focused exercises, which are ordered based on their difficulty: beginner, intermediate, and advanced (see Table 1.1). They each contain a brief overview of the exercise, examples of client–therapist interactions to help guide trainees, step-by-step instructions for conducting that exercise, and a list of criteria for mastering the relevant skill. The client statements and sample therapist responses are then presented, also organized by difficulty. The statements and responses are presented separately so that the trainee playing the therapist has more freedom to improvise responses without being influenced by the sample responses, which should only be used if the trainee has difficulty improvising their own responses. Exercise 7 follows a different format than the other exercises, using back-and-forth, client–therapist dialogues instead of a single client statement followed by a single response.

The last two exercises in Part II provide opportunities to practice the 10 skills within simulated psychotherapy sessions. Exercise 11 provides a sample psychotherapy session transcript in which the IPT skills are used and clearly labeled, thereby demonstrating how they might flow together in an actual therapy session. IPT trainees are invited to run through the sample transcript, with one playing the therapist and the other playing the client, to get a feel for how a session might unfold. Exercise 12 provides suggestions for undertaking mock sessions, as well as client profiles ordered by difficulty (beginner, intermediate, and advanced) that trainees can use for improvised role-plays.

Part III contains Chapter 3, which provides additional guidance for trainers and trainees. While Chapter 2 is more procedural, Chapter 3 covers big-picture issues. It highlights six key points for getting the most out of deliberate practice and describes the importance of appropriate responsiveness, attending to trainee well-being and respecting their privacy, and trainer self-evaluation, among other topics.

Four appendixes conclude this book. Appendix A provides instructions for monitoring and adjusting the difficulty of each exercise as needed. It provides a Deliberate Practice Reaction Form for the trainee playing the therapist to complete to indicate whether the exercise is too easy or too difficult. Appendix B includes a Deliberate Practice Diary Form that can be used during a training session's final evaluation to process the trainees' experiences, but its primary purpose is to provide trainees a format to explore and record their experiences while engaging in additional, between-session deliberate practice activities without the supervisor. Appendix C presents additional approaches and guidelines for troubleshooting the implementation of the Interpersonal Inventory in Exercise 2. Appendix D presents a sample syllabus demonstrating how the 10 deliberate practice exercises and other support material can be integrated into a wider IPT training course. Instructors may choose to modify the syllabus or pick elements of it to integrate into their own courses.

Downloadable versions of this book's appendixes, including a color version of the Deliberate Practice Reaction Form, can be found in the "Resources" tab online (https://www.apa.org/pubs/books/deliberate-practice-interpersonal-psychotherapy).

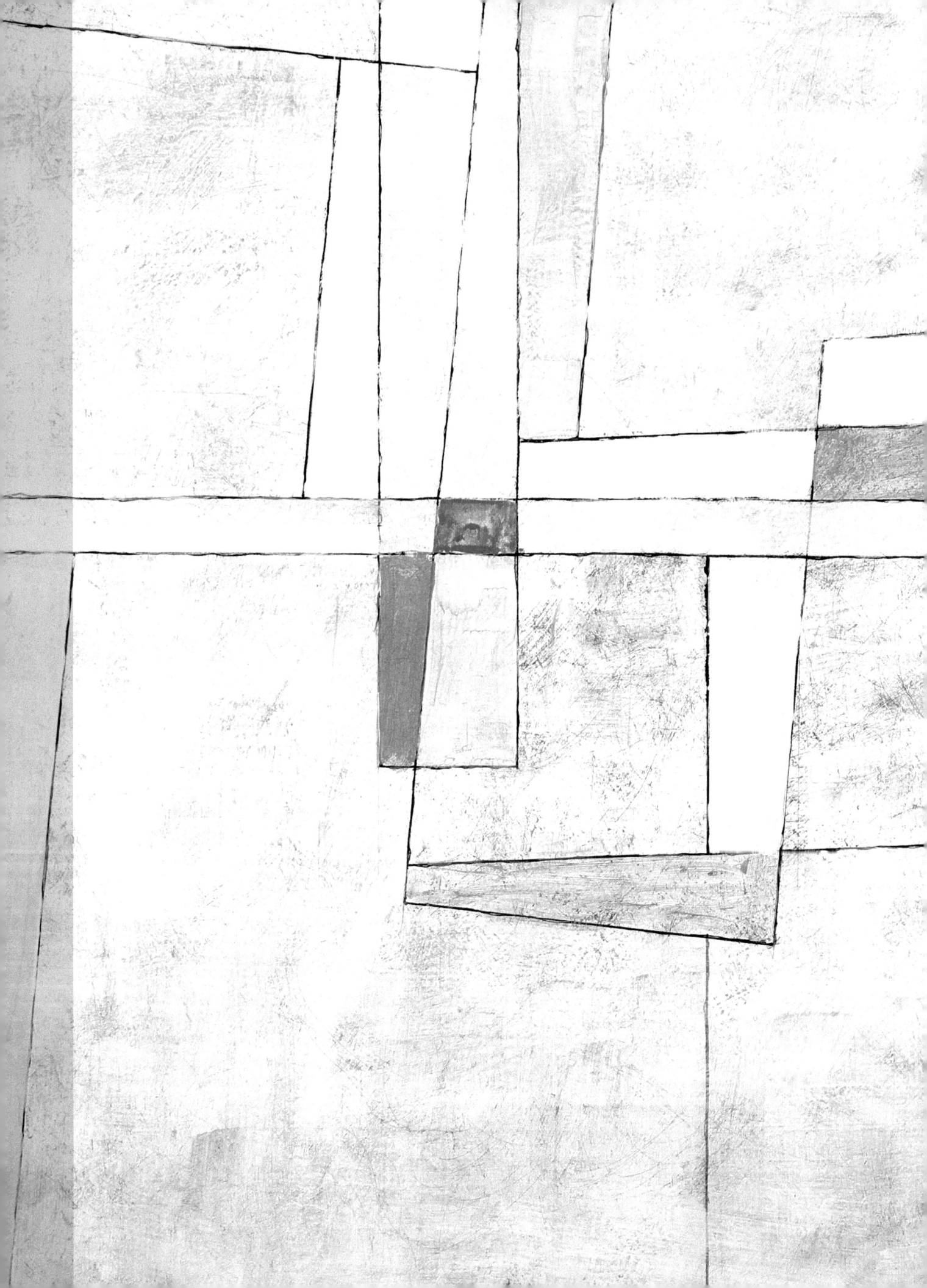

Instructions for the Interpersonal Psychotherapy Deliberate Practice Exercises

This chapter provides basic instructions that are common to all the exercises in this book. More specific instructions are provided in each exercise. Chapter 3 also provides important guidance for trainees and trainers that will help them get the most out of deliberate practice. Appendix A offers additional instructions for monitoring and adjusting the difficulty of the exercises as needed after getting through all then client statements in a single difficulty level, including a Deliberate Practice Reaction Form the trainee playing the therapist can complete to indicate whether they found the statements too easy or too difficult. **Difficulty assessment is an important part of the deliberate practice process and should not be skipped.**

Overview

The deliberate practice exercises in this book involve role-plays of hypothetical situations in therapy. The role-play involves three people: one trainee role-plays the therapist, another trainee role-plays the client, and a trainer (professor/supervisor) observes and provides feedback. Alternately, a peer can observe and provide feedback.

This book provides a script for each role-play, each with a client statement and also with an example therapist response. The client statements are graded in difficulty from beginning to advanced, although these difficulty grades are only estimates. The actual perceived difficulty of client statements is subjective and varies widely by trainee. For example, some trainees may experience a stimulus of a client being angry to be easy to respond to, whereas another trainee may experience it as very difficult. Thus, it is important for trainees to provide difficulty assessments and adjustments to ensure that they are practicing at the right difficulty level: neither too easy nor too hard.

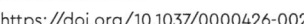

https://doi.org/10.1037/0000426-002

Deliberate Practice in Interpersonal Psychotherapy, by O. Belik, J. M. Schultz, S. Fairhurst, S. Stuart, A. Vaz, and T. Rousmaniere

Time Frame

We recommend a 90-minute time block for every exercise, structured roughly as follows:

- First 20 minutes: Orientation. The trainer explains the interpersonal psychotherapy (IPT) skill and demonstrates the exercise procedure with a volunteer trainee.

- Middle 50 minutes: Trainees perform the exercise in pairs. The trainer or a peer provides feedback throughout this process and monitors/adjusts the exercise's difficulty as needed after each set of statements (see Appendix A for more information about difficulty assessment).

- Final 20 minutes: Review, feedback, and discussion.

Preparation

1. Every trainee will need their own copy of this book.

2. Each exercise requires the trainer to fill out a Deliberate Practice Reaction Form after completing all the statements from a single difficulty level. This form is available in the "Resources" tab online (https://www.apa.org/pubs/books/deliberate-practice-interpersonal-psychotherapy) and in Appendix A.

3. Trainees are grouped into pairs. One volunteers to role-play the therapist and one to role-play the client (they will switch roles after 15 minutes of practice). As noted previously, an observer who might be either the trainer or a fellow trainee will work with each pair.

The Role of the Trainer

The primary responsibilities of the trainer are as follows:

1. Provide corrective feedback, which includes both information about how well the trainees' response met expected criteria and any necessary guidance about how to improve the response.

2. Remind trainees to do difficulty assessments and adjustments after each level of client statements is completed (beginning, intermediate, and advanced).

How to Practice

Each exercise includes its own step-by-step instructions. Trainees should follow these instructions carefully, as every step is important.

Skill Criteria

Each of the first 10 exercises focuses on one essential IPT skill with skill criteria that describe the important components or principles for that skill.

The goal of the role-play is for trainees to practice improvising responses to the client statement in a manner that (a) is attuned to the client, (b) meets skill criteria as much as possible, and (c) feels authentic for the trainee. Trainees are provided scripts with example therapist responses to give them a sense of how to incorporate the skill criteria into a response. **It is important, however, that trainees do not read the example responses verbatim in the role-plays!** Therapy is highly personal and improvisational; the goal of deliberate practice is to develop trainees' ability to improvise within a consistent framework. Memorizing scripted responses would be counterproductive for helping trainees learn to perform therapy that is responsive, authentic, and attuned to each individual client.

The book's authors wrote the scripted example responses. However, trainees' personal style of therapy may differ slightly or greatly from that in the example scripts. It is essential that, over time, trainees develop their own style and voice, while simultaneously being able to intervene according to the model's principles and strategies. To facilitate this, the exercises in this book were designed to maximize opportunities for improvisational responses informed by the skill criteria and ongoing feedback.

The goal for the role-plays is for trainees to practice improvising responses to the client statements in a manner that is

- attuned to the client,
- meets as many of the skill criteria as possible, and
- feels authentic for the trainee.

Review, Feedback, and Discussion

The review and feedback sequence after each role-play has these two elements:

- First, the trainee who played the client **briefly** shares how it felt to be on the receiving end of the therapist response. This can help assess how well trainees are attuning with the client.

- Second, the trainer provides **brief** feedback (less than 1 minute) based on the skill criteria for each exercise. Keep feedback specific, behavioral, and brief to preserve time for skill rehearsal. If one trainer is teaching multiple pairs of trainees, the trainer walks around the room, observing the pairs and offering brief feedback. When the trainer is not available, the trainee playing the client gives peer feedback to the therapist, based on the skill criteria and how it felt to be on the receiving end of the intervention. Alternately, a third trainee can observe and provide feedback.

Trainers (or peers) should remember to keep all feedback specific and brief and not to veer into discussions of theory. There are many other settings for extended discussion of IPT theory and research. In deliberate practice, it is of utmost importance to maximize time for continuous behavioral rehearsal via role-plays.

Final Evaluation

After both trainees have role-played the client and the therapist, the trainer provides an evaluation. Participants should engage in a short group discussion based on this evaluation. This discussion can provide ideas for where to focus homework and future deliberate practice sessions. To this end, Appendix B presents a Deliberate Practice Diary Form, which can also be downloaded from the "Resources" tab online (https://www. apa.org/pubs/books/deliberate-practice-interpersonal-psychotherapy). This form can be used by trainees as a template to help them explore and record their experiences of deliberate practice activities between focused training sessions with a supervisor.

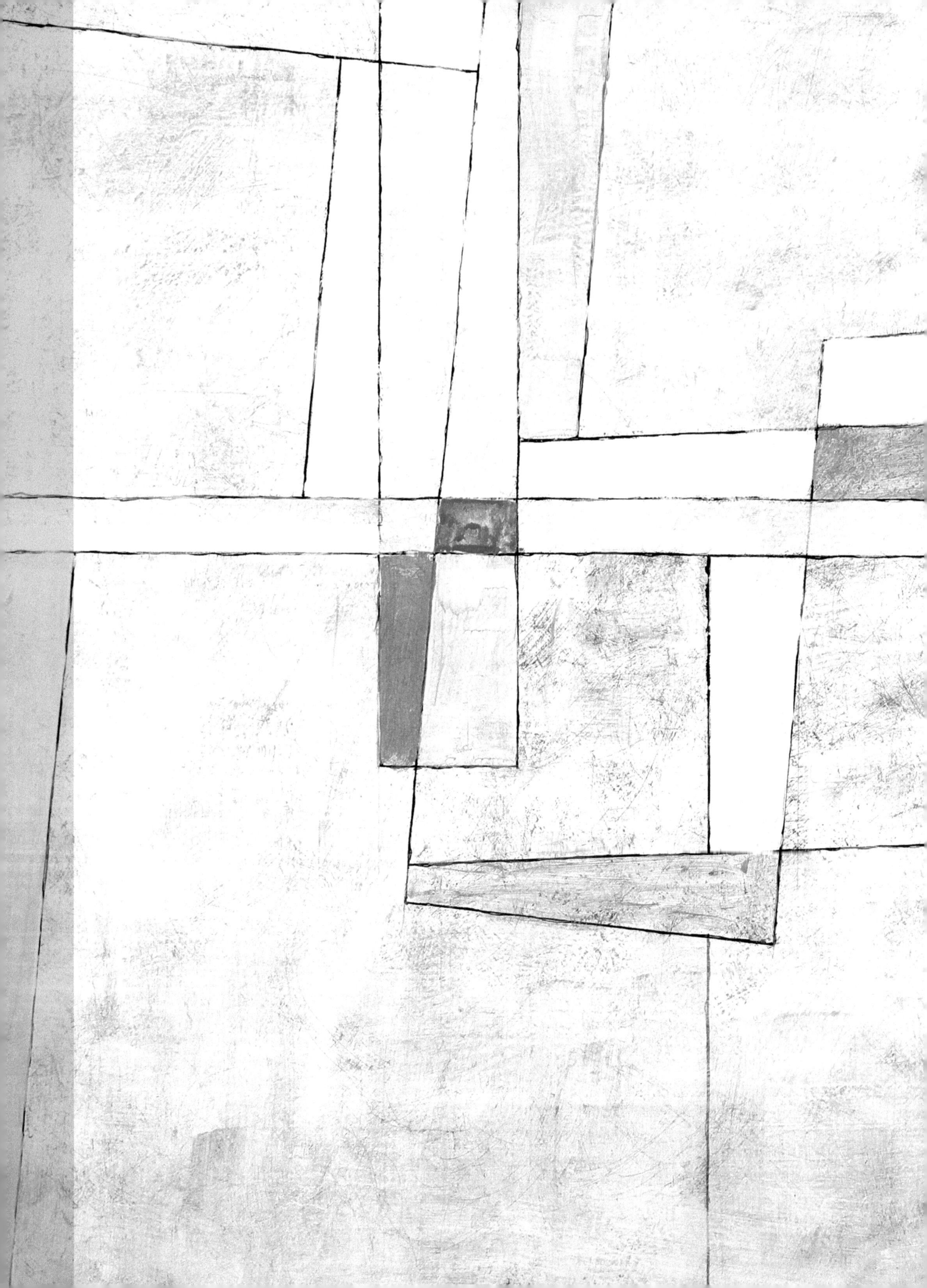

Deliberate Practice Exercises for Interpersonal Psychotherapy Skills

This section of the book provides 10 deliberate practice exercises for essential interpersonal psychotherapy (IPT) skills. These exercises are organized in a developmental sequence, from those that are appropriate for someone just beginning IPT training to exercises for those who have progressed to a more advanced level. Although we anticipate that most trainers will use these exercises in the order we have suggested, some trainers may find it more appropriate for their training circumstances to use a different order. We also provide two comprehensive exercises that bring together the IPT skills using an annotated IPT session transcript and mock sessions.

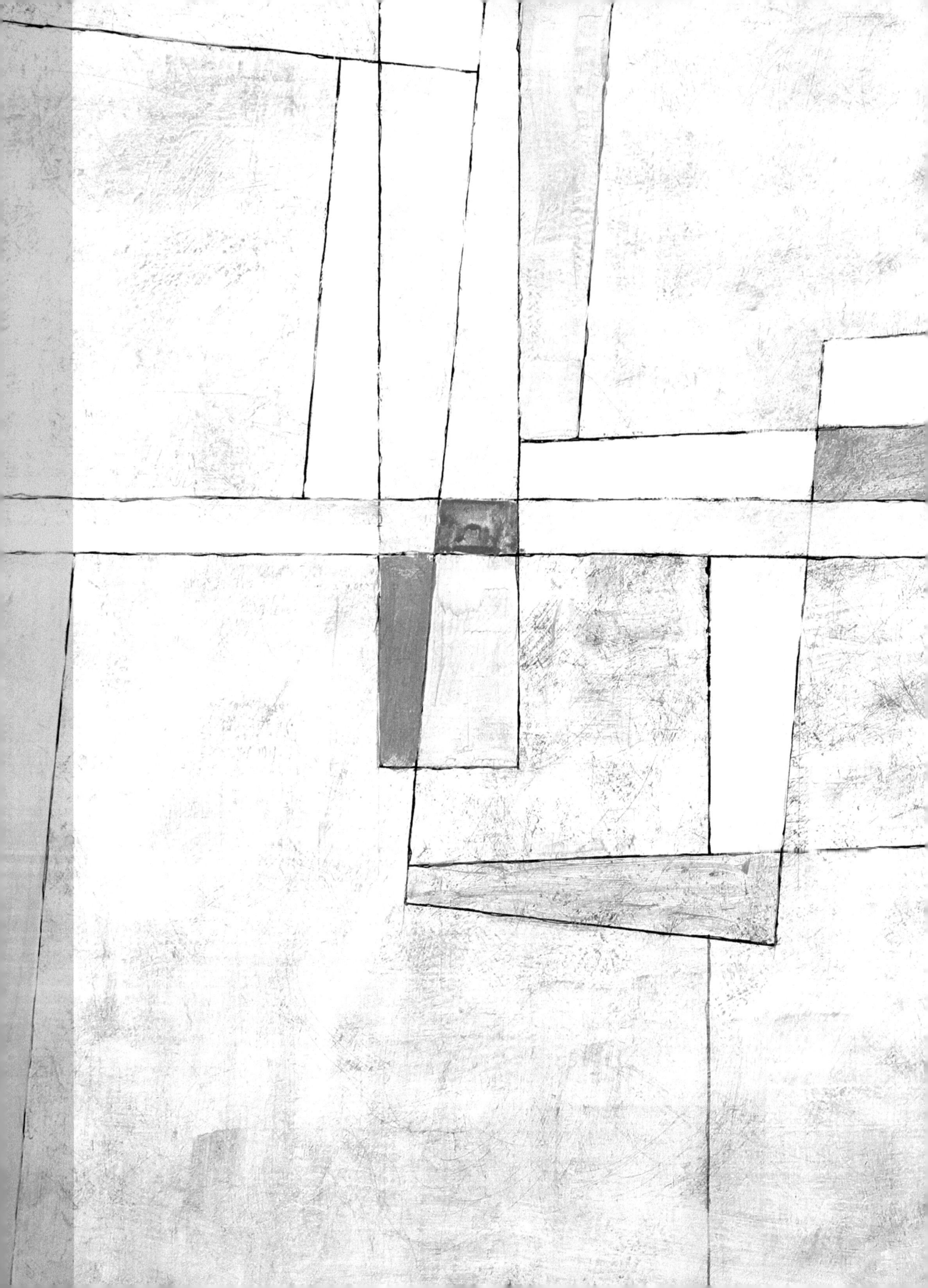

Presenting the Interpersonal Inventory: Interpersonal Inventory I

Preparations for Exercise 1

1. Read the instructions in Chapter 2.

2. Download the Deliberate Practice Reaction Form and the Deliberate Practice Diary Form at https://www.apa.org/pubs/books/deliberate-practice-interpersonal-psychotherapy (see the "Resources" tab; also available in Appendixes A and B, respectively).

Skill Description

Skill Difficulty Level: Beginner

Interpersonal psychotherapy (IPT) is designed to improve clients' interpersonal distress. This is facilitated by increasing clients' communication skills and improving their social support. Cocreating an Interpersonal Inventory is therefore a unique and critical intervention in IPT because it allows the clinician to gather information efficiently about the clients' social support system, including the quality of support and typical interactions within specific relationships. It is an overview or a bird's-eye view of the client's social support network and includes family, friends, and people in their community. The inventory is an integral and defining element of IPT.

The Interpersonal Inventory or "Circle" is usually constructed in Session 2 of IPT after a comprehensive intake in Session 1. The cocreation of the inventory starts with the therapist drawing two concentric circles. The inner circle (the donut hole) represents the client's "intimate" support circle, and the middle ring (the donut itself) represents their "close" supports. The outer area represents "extended" or more distant individuals. An example of a completed Interpersonal Inventory is depicted in Figure E1.1.

https://doi.org/10.1037/0000426-003

Deliberate Practice in Interpersonal Psychotherapy, by O. Belik, J. M. Schultz, S. Fairhurst, S. Stuart, A. Vaz, and T. Rousmaniere

FIGURE E1.1. Example of a Completed Interpersonal Inventory

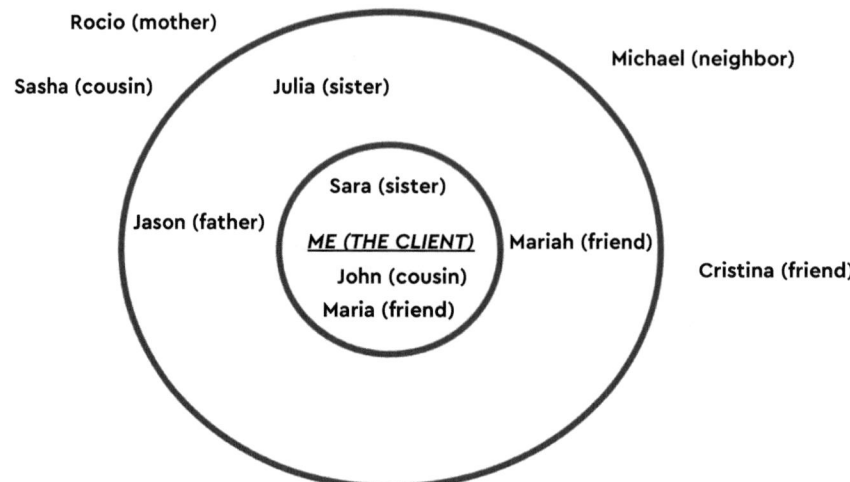

It is critical to note that the point of the inventory is simply to assess social support. It is designed to get a general sense of the client's relationships—a baseline from which to work. Because IPT is based on attachment theory and the concept of relational frame, understanding the client's relationships and the support others do or do not provide is critical. This information will be used to determine which relationships are problematic and need to be addressed in the middle phase of IPT, and which provide support that the client can learn to elicit.

It is also important to note that there are no right or wrong answers when coconstructing an inventory. The point is to gain a better understanding of the client's perspective about their relationships. Collaborating to collect this information in an open and nonjudgmental way provides insight into the client's expectations and hopes for their relationships, information about their communication style, attachment style, and relational difficulties that may be contributing to or maintaining their interpersonal distress.

The simplicity of the Interpersonal Circle is part of its appeal. It is very to explain, use, and work with—so much so that the client can fill it out. Having the client do so, in collaboration with the therapist, ultimately leads to obtaining much better information. To achieve this, the client should be the one writing the names of people who do or do not support them on the diagram. Later, once the client has put the names on the Circle diagram, the therapist can ask follow-up questions about the various relationships. This information will help understand in detail what the client's support system is actually like.

The therapist's introduction of the inventory is a critical skill because it sets the tone for the therapy and helps establish a collaborative relationship. The request from the therapist—and it is a request, not a demand, for the client to do a task—should be an invitation to the client to help the clinician better understand what the client's relationships are like. Modeling good communication will be a tool the therapist can use throughout IPT to help clients learn to improve their own communication.

The therapist should improvise a response to each patient statement following the following skill criteria:

1. **Present the plan for the session, which is to conduct the Interpersonal Inventory.** The therapist starts by explicitly making a request to cocreate an inventory with the client. Doing so provides direction and structure to the therapy session. A typical introduction to this might be "Today I would like to invite you to complete an Interpersonal Inventory."

2. **Present a rationale for the use of the Interpersonal Inventory.** It is important to communicate that the Interpersonal Inventory is a way for the therapist and client to gain a better understanding of the different types and quality of support the client is or is not getting from different people in their life. This will help better understand, use, and improve the client's social support during the course of therapy. A typical presentation of this might be "The Inventory, or Circle, is a way to help us both understand what your relationships with the important people in your life are like."

3. **Present the design and the definitions of circles.** After presenting the rationale for constructing the inventory, the therapist then draws the inventory diagram (i.e., two concentric circles that represent the client's social support; see Figure 1.5 in Chapter 1) and explains the task they will engage in together. A typical explanation of how to do so might be as follows: "I'd like you to write the names of seven to 10 people who are important to you. In the inner circle, you can write your 'intimate' supports—people who provide you with a great deal of support. The one right outside of that should include your 'close support' people, those that are important but not quite so close or supportive, and the rest of the space would include your 'extended' supports, people who are more distant. There are no right or wrong answers, and you can include anyone you'd like. What I am interested in is your perspective."

4. **Check in to see if the client has any questions.** It is good practice in IPT to check in with the client after every set of instructions regarding a therapeutic task. This is an essential part of IPT because it fosters good communication within the therapeutic relationship and models good communication for the client so that they can learn to use similar communication in their relationships outside of therapy as well. A typical check-in might be as follows: "Do you have any questions about what we are doing and why?"

SKILL CRITERIA FOR EXERCISE 1

1. Present the plan for the session to conduct the Interpersonal Inventory.
2. Present a rationale for the use of the Interpersonal Inventory.
3. Present the design and the definitions of circles.
4. Check in to ask if the client has any questions.

Examples of Therapists Presenting the Interpersonal Inventory

Example 1

CLIENT: [*upbeat*] I've been looking forward to this session. The last one seemed more like just getting a history. Where should we start?

THERAPIST: That's great to hear! Today I would like to invite you to complete what we call an Interpersonal Inventory. (Criterion 1) The inventory is a way for us to understand the different levels of support you get from different people in your life. This will help us better understand, use, and improve your social support as we work together. (Criterion 2) I'm going to draw two circles, and then I'd like for you to write the names of seven to 10 people who are important to you on the diagram. In the inner circle you can put your "intimate" supports, the one right outside of that should include your "close support" people, and the rest of the space should include your "extended" supports. There are no right or wrong answers; you can write down people wherever you like. (Criterion 3) Do you have any questions about what we are doing? (Criterion 4)

Example 2

CLIENT: [*unsure*] I am not sure where to start the session today.

THERAPIST: Good question. Today we can start with what we call an Interpersonal Inventory. (Criterion 1) The Interpersonal Inventory is a way for us to understand the different levels of support you have from different people in your life. This will help us better understand your relationships, and later to use and improve your social support as we work together. (Criterion 2) I'm going to draw two circles: The one in the middle will be your "intimate" support circle, one right after that one is "close support," and the rest of the space could represent "extended" support. Please write down the names of seven to 10 people where you think they would best be placed. (Criterion 3) Do you have any questions about anything I've said so far? (Criterion 4)

Example 3

CLIENT: [*engaged*] What do you want us to talk about in session today?

THERAPIST: Today we can start working on what we call an Interpersonal Inventory. (Criterion 1) The Interpersonal Inventory is a way for us both to understand the different levels of support you have from different people in your life. This will help us better understand those relationships, and later use and improve your social supports as we work together. (Criterion 2) I am going to draw two circles: The one in the middle will be your "intimate" support circle, the next one out are your "close supports," and the rest of the space could represent your "extended" supports. (Criterion 3) Do you have any questions about anything I've said so far? (Criterion 4)

INSTRUCTIONS FOR EXERCISE 1

Step 1: Role-Play and Feedback

- The client says the first beginner client statement. The therapist then **improvises** a response based on the skill criteria.
- The trainer (or, if not available, the client) provides **brief** feedback based on the skill criteria.
- The client then repeats the same statement, and the therapist again improvises a response. The trainer (or client) again provides brief feedback.

Step 2: Repeat

- Repeat Step 1 for all the statements **in the current difficulty level** (beginner, intermediate, or advanced).

Step 3: Assess and Adjust Difficulty

- The therapist completes the Deliberate Practice Reaction Form (see Appendix A) and decides whether to make the exercise easier or harder or to repeat the same difficulty level.

Step 4: Repeat for Approximately 15 Minutes

- Repeat Steps 1 to 3 for at least 15 minutes.
- The trainees then switch therapist and client roles and start over.

Now it's your turn! Follow Steps 1 and 2 from the exercise instructions.

Remember: The goal of the role-play is for trainees to practice improvising responses to the client statements in a manner that (a) uses the skill criteria and (b) feels authentic for the trainee. **Example therapist responses for each client statement are provided at the end of this exercise. Trainees should attempt to improvise their own responses before reading the examples.**

BEGINNER-LEVEL CLIENT STATEMENTS FOR EXERCISE 1
Beginner Client Statement 1
[Eager] I thought about our last session and want to continue to talk about my family and friends. Is that OK?
Beginner Client Statement 2
[Excited] I have made a new friend at school today and wanted to talk about it.
Beginner Client Statement 3
[Tearful] Ever since I moved here, I feel lonely and do not have enough friends in my life.
Beginner Client Statement 4
[Upbeat] I have been feeling excited to see you! I want to continue talking about my coworker I mentioned last session.
Beginner Client Statement 5
[Sad] I miss my friend who moved away a couple of weeks ago and don't know who to reach out to for support.

 Assess and adjust the difficulty before moving to the next difficulty level (see Step 3 in the exercise instructions).

INTERMEDIATE-LEVEL CLIENT STATEMENTS FOR EXERCISE 1
Intermediate Client Statement 1
[Sad] I'm not sure what to talk about today. I have been feeling sad.
Intermediate Client Statement 2
[Thoughtful] I have been feeling disconnected from people lately. What do you think I should do?
Intermediate Client Statement 3
[Engaged] I know I ask a lot of questions here, but how can I make friends who care about me?
Intermediate Client Statement 4
[Neutral] I think I feel OK today, nothing is really bothering me. What do you think we should talk about?
Intermediate Client Statement 5
[Upbeat] I'm so glad we have a session today! I need to talk about my relationship with my brother.

🛑 **Assess and adjust the difficulty before moving to the next difficulty level (see Step 3 in the exercise instructions).**

ADVANCED-LEVEL CLIENT STATEMENTS FOR EXERCISE 1
Advanced Client Statement 1
[Frustrated] I have so many people around me, but I don't feel like they understand me.
Advanced Client Statement 2
[Upset] I had a fight with one of my friends today and my other friends are on his side. I don't think I talked about him or my other friends yet . . . can I tell you about them?
Advanced Client Statement 3
[Angry] I don't feel that my boss is supportive of me. I am not sure if I actually have anyone who supports me at work. . . . **[Sad]** Why do you think that is?
Advanced Client Statement 4
[Thoughtful] I feel like I keep giving and giving and giving to other people and don't really feel supported in return. When I think about it, I feel sad and tired. . . . And don't really want to help other people anymore.
Advanced Client Statement 5
[Sad] I went to a party last weekend and realized that I don't really feel close to some of my "friends." . . . And I started to feel sad. . . . Maybe I need new friends, what do you think?

Assess and adjust the difficulty here (see Step 3 in the exercise instructions). If appropriate, follow the instructions to make the exercise even more challenging (see Appendix A).

Example Therapist Responses: Presenting the Interpersonal Inventory

Remember: Trainees should attempt to improvise their own responses before reading the example responses. **Do not read the following responses verbatim unless you are having trouble coming up with your own!**

EXAMPLE RESPONSES TO BEGINNER-LEVEL CLIENT STATEMENTS FOR EXERCISE 1
Example Response to Beginner Client Statement 1
I am glad you thought about our last session and today, as a way to talk about your family and friends, I would like to invite you to complete what we call an Interpersonal Inventory. (Criterion 1) The Interpersonal Inventory is a very specific way to look at your social support—your family, your friends, and other people in your life. It will help us to take an "inventory" of your social milieu and allow us to better understand your relationships. (Criterion 2) To start the Interpersonal Inventory, I'll draw two circles: The one in the center will be your "intimate" support circle, the second one will be your "close supports," and the rest of the space that is left could represent "extended" support. I'd like you to write down the names of seven to 10 people on the diagram, placing them where it makes sense to you. (Criterion 3) How does that sound to you? Do you have any questions about anything I've said so far? (Criterion 4)
Example Response to Beginner Client Statement 2
I am so glad to hear that you have made a new friend at school, relationships matter so much! I would love to talk about your new friend and the other people in your life. One way to do it would be to complete what we call an Interpersonal Inventory. (Criterion 1) The Interpersonal Inventory is a unique way to create a "visual" picture of the important people in your life and the levels of support that they provide to you. This will help us understand the different relationships you have with people in your life. It will also help us figure out how to use and improve your social support. (Criterion 2) Let me start by drawing two circles: The first one in the middle will be your "intimate" support circle, the next one around it will be your "close supports," and the rest of the space could represent your "extended" supports. I'd like you to write down the names of 10 or so people, placing them on the diagram where it makes sense to you. (Criterion 3) Do you have any questions about anything I've said so far? (Criterion 4)
Example Response to Beginner Client Statement 3
Oh, I see and feel how sad you are feeling. Sometimes moving away from people and places you know can bring a sense of grief and sadness. As you are adjusting and getting to know new people in your life, it might be helpful for us to look at old connections that you are maintaining with people and new people who are entering your life. A good way to look at the relationships in your life is to create what we call an Interpersonal Inventory. (Criterion 1) The Interpersonal Inventory is a way for us to see who is in your life and the different kinds of support you have from them. It will also allow us to explore who might be missing. This will help us better understand your feelings of "loneliness" and eventually use and improve your social support as we work together. (Criterion 2) I am going to draw two circles: The one in the middle will be your "intimate" support circle, the next one out should include your "close supports," and the rest of the space could represent your "extended" supports. Please write the names of eight to 10 people on the diagram where you think that they should go. (Criterion 3) Do you have any questions about what we are going to do? (Criterion 4)

EXAMPLE RESPONSES TO BEGINNER-LEVEL CLIENT STATEMENTS FOR EXERCISE 1

Example Response to Beginner Client Statement 4

I am glad to see you as well, and today we can continue to discuss different people in your life, including your coworker. To do this, it would be helpful to look at your relationship with your coworker as well as at other people in your life. We can do that by completing what we call an Interpersonal Inventory. (Criterion 1) The Interpersonal Inventory is a way for us to look at different people in your life all at once, while understanding the unique place that each relationship holds for you. This will help us better understand the different relational needs you have and how they are being met right now. (Criterion 2) I'm going to draw two circles: The one in the middle will include your "intimate" support circle, the one right after should include your "close supports," and the rest of the space could represent your "extended" supports. (Criterion 3) Do you have any questions about anything I've said so far? (Criterion 4)

Example Response to Beginner Client Statement 5

[Leaning forward a bit] I see how sad you are, missing your friend. I am thinking it might be helpful to look at the support you currently have in your life, including the connection with your friend who moved away. One way to do that is to complete what we call an Interpersonal Inventory. (Criterion 1) The Interpersonal Inventory is a way for us to think about and list the important people in your life. Some might be closer to you, and some might feel further away, but they are still present in your life. We can look at the different levels of support that might be available to you from people in your life. (Criterion 2) I'm going to draw two circles: The one in the middle will be your "intimate" support circle, the one right after can be your "close supports," and the rest of the space could represent your "extended" supports. Please write down the names of eight to 10 people who are important to you; you can put them wherever seems best to you. (Criterion 3) Do you have any questions about anything I've said so far? (Criterion 4)

EXAMPLE RESPONSES TO INTERMEDIATE-LEVEL CLIENT STATEMENTS FOR EXERCISE 1

Example Response to Intermediate Client Statement 1

Yes, I feel sadness in your voice and would like to offer you some guidance about how we can start the session today, if it's OK with you. I am wondering if it would be helpful to continue to talk about different relationships in your life so that we can better understand your support system and the emotional impact your social connections have on you. In interpersonal psychotherapy, there is a helpful way to look at your social support, which is to construct what we call an Interpersonal Inventory. (Criterion 1) The Interpersonal Inventory is a way for us to understand the different levels of support you have from different people in your life. This will help us to better understand them, and later use and improve your social support as we work together. (Criterion 2) I'm going to draw two circles: The one in the middle will be your "intimate" support circle, one right outside of that will be for "close supports," and the rest of the space could represent your "extended" supports. (Criterion 3) Do you have any questions about anything I've said so far? (Criterion 4)

Example Response to Intermediate Client Statement 2

I see. You know, it might be helpful to take some time to understand the people who are in your life and thus to start understanding what makes you feel disconnected. We can talk about who you feel closer to and who you feel disconnected from. One way to approach this is to complete what we call an Interpersonal Inventory. (Criterion 1) The Interpersonal Inventory is a way for us to better understand the different degrees of closeness you have with people in your life. This will help us to start discovering what helps you to feel closer to other people and what contributes to your feeling of "disconnect." (Criterion 2) I'm going to draw two circles: The one in the middle will be your "intimate" support circle, one right after that one is "close support," and the rest of the space could represent "extended" support. You can write down the names of eight or more people on the circles where you think they should go. (Criterion 3) Do you have any questions about how we are going to do this? (Criterion 4)

Example Response to Intermediate Client Statement 3

Good question. It might be helpful for us first to start understanding who the people in your life are that you currently consider to be friends. To do this, I'd like to invite you to complete what we call an Interpersonal Inventory. (Criterion 1) The Interpersonal Inventory is a way for us both to understand the different levels of support you have from different people in your life. This will help us better understand those relationships, and then later, use and improve your social support as we work together. (Criterion 2) I'm going to draw two circles: The one in the center will be your "intimate" support circle, the one outside of that one is for your "close supports," and the rest of the space could represent your "extended" supports. You can write down around 10 or so people on the diagram where you wish. (Criterion 3) Any questions about anything I've said so far? (Criterion 4)

Example Response to Intermediate Client Statement 4

I am glad to hear that you feel OK today, so I would like to invite you to complete what we call an Interpersonal Inventory. (Criterion 1) The Interpersonal Inventory is a way for us to understand the different levels of support you have from different people in your life. This will help us better understand those relationships, and later we can work on how to use and improve your social support to get the help you need. (Criterion 2) I'm going to draw a donut that you can write on. The donut hole will be your "intimate" support circle, the actual donut part is for your "close supports," and the space around the donut represents your "extended" supports. (Criterion 3) Do you have any questions about anything I've said so far? (Criterion 4)

EXAMPLE RESPONSES TO INTERMEDIATE-LEVEL
CLIENT STATEMENTS FOR EXERCISE 1

Example Response to Intermediate Client Statement 5

Yes, I'm glad you came to the session too. We can talk about your relationship with your brother and other people in your life; in fact, I would like to invite you to complete what we call an Interpersonal Inventory to do just that. (Criterion 1) The Interpersonal Inventory is a way for us to understand the different levels of support you have from different people in your life. This will help us better understand, use, and improve your social support as we work together. (Criterion 2) I'm going to draw what looks like a bagel. The hole in the middle is to represent your "intimate" support circle, the bagel part is for your "close supports," and the rest of the space outside the bagel represents your "extended" supports. You can write down the names of seven to 10 people where you think they should go. (Criterion 3) Do you have any questions about anything I've said so far? (Criterion 4)

EXAMPLE RESPONSES TO ADVANCED-LEVEL CLIENT STATEMENTS FOR EXERCISE 1

Example Response to Advanced Client Statement 1

I can see how frustrated you are. It might be helpful to first understand who you have in your life and then see what your relationships are like and the kinds of support you receive from different people. To do that I would like to invite you to complete what we call an Interpersonal Inventory. (Criterion 1) The Interpersonal Inventory is a way for us to understand the different levels of support you have from people in your life. This will help us better understand, and eventually use and improve, your social support as we work together. (Criterion 2) I'm going to draw two circles with one inside of the other: The one in the very middle will be your "intimate" support circle, the one outside of that one is for your "close supports," and the rest of the space could represent your "extended" support relationships. Please write down the names of seven to 10 people depending on how much support you get from them—no right or wrong answers. (Criterion 3) Do you have any questions about anything I've said so far? (Criterion 4)

Example Response to Advanced Client Statement 2

I hear you are upset about the situation and yes, I agree—it might be helpful for us to start by talking about your friends and other people in your life. Today I would like to invite you to complete what we call an Interpersonal Inventory. (Criterion 1) The Interpersonal Inventory is a way for us to understand the different levels of support you have from different people in your life. This will help us better understand, and eventually use and improve, your social support as we work together. (Criterion 2) I'm going to draw two circles: The one in the middle will be your "intimate" support circle, the one right after that is for your "close support" people, and the rest of the space is for your "extended" support people. Please write down the names of seven to 10 people and put them where you think they best fit—no right or wrong answers. (Criterion 3) Do you have any questions about anything I've said so far? (Criterion 4)

Example Response to Advanced Client Statement 3

Oh, that does sound tiring to keep giving support to people without feeling supported in return. To understand more what that is like for you, I am thinking it might be helpful to complete what we call an Interpersonal Inventory. (Criterion 1) The Interpersonal Inventory is a written tool we can use to understand the different levels of support you have from different people in your life. This will help us better understand those relationships, and eventually to help you use and improve your social support as we work together. (Criterion 2) I'm going to draw two circles: The one in the middle will be your "intimate" support circle, one right after that one is your "close supports," and the rest of the space could represent your "extended" support people. (Criterion 3) Do you have any questions about anything I've said so far? (Criterion 4)

Example Response to Advanced Client Statement 4

Your thoughts make a lot of sense. What would help in this area is for us to complete what we call an Interpersonal Inventory. (Criterion 1) The Interpersonal Inventory is a way for us to understand the different levels of support you have from different people in your life. It will help us better understand how those relationships work, and then to use and improve your social support as we work together in therapy. (Criterion 2) After I draw the diagram for you, I'd like you to write down the names of seven to 10 people and put them on the diagram based on the quality of support you get from them. There are two circles: The center one should include your "intimate" supports, the middle one is for "close supports," and the rest of the space is for your "extended" supports. (Criterion 3) Do you have any questions about anything I've said so far? (Criterion 4)

**EXAMPLE RESPONSES TO ADVANCED-LEVEL
CLIENT STATEMENTS FOR EXERCISE 1**

Example Response to Advanced Client Statement 5

I can see you are feeling sad, and I am wondering if it might be helpful for us to talk about different people in your life, including your family and friends, and how they are affecting your mood and distress. To do that, I'd like to invite you to complete what we call an Interpersonal Inventory. (Criterion 1) The Interpersonal Inventory is a way for us to understand the different levels of support you have from different people in your life. This will help us better understand, and eventually use and improve, your social support as we work together. (Criterion 2) I'm drawing two circles: The one in the middle is your "intimate" support circle, the one right outside of that is for your "close supports," and the rest of the space is for your "extended" support relationships. You can write down nine or 10 people and put them where you think they best fit—no right or wrong answers. (Criterion 3) Do you have any questions about anything I've said so far? (Criterion 4)

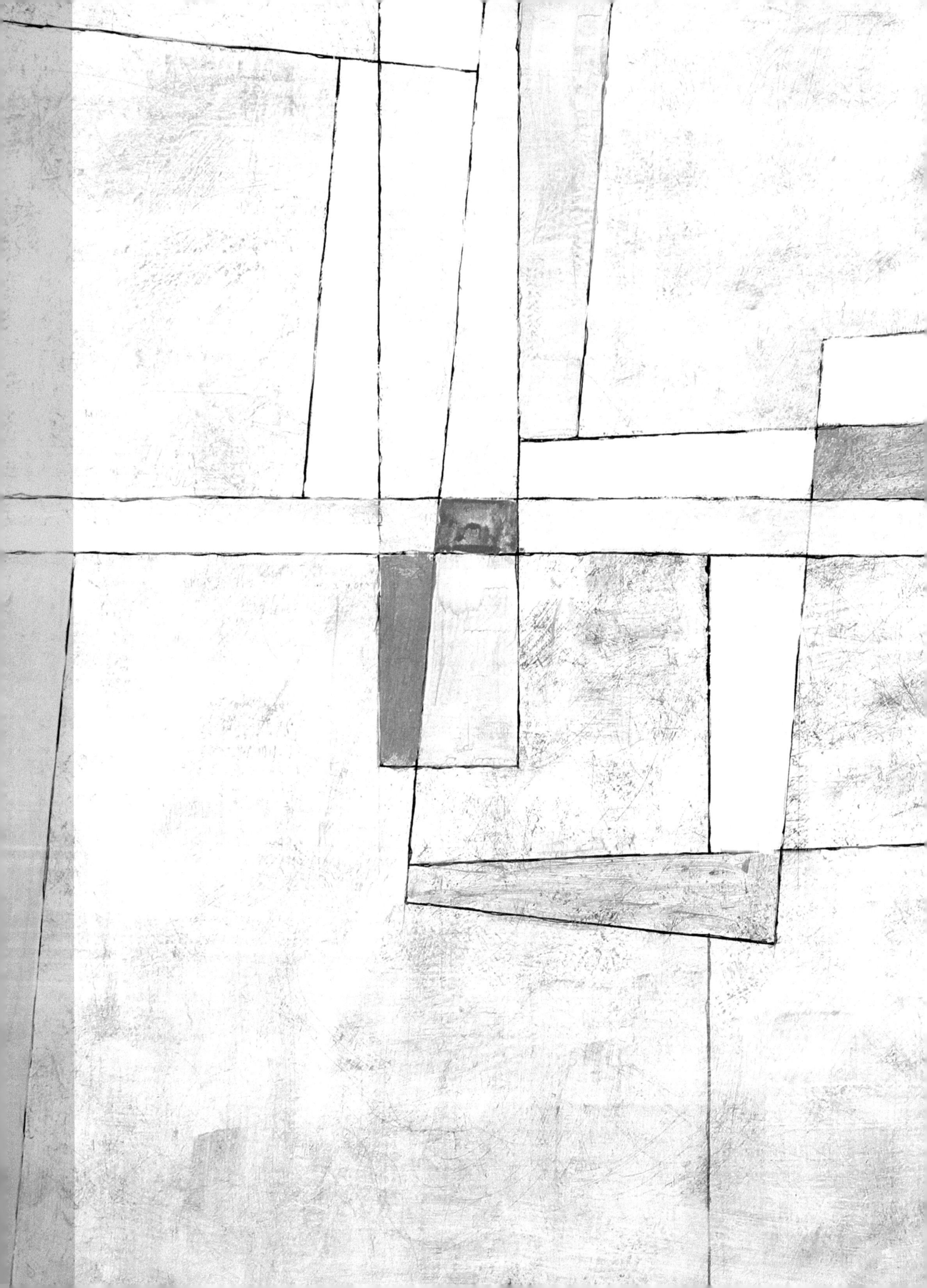

Exploring Interpersonal Relationships: Interpersonal Inventory II

Preparations for Exercise 2

1. Read the instructions in Chapter 2.

2. Download the Deliberate Practice Reaction Form and the Deliberate Practice Diary Form at https://www.apa.org/pubs/books/deliberate-practice-interpersonal-psychotherapy (see the "Resources" tab; also available in Appendixes A and B, respectively).

Skill Description

Skill Difficulty Level: Beginner

As described in Exercise 1, the Interpersonal Inventory is a critical intervention that is unique to interpersonal psychotherapy (IPT). It allows the clinician and the client to understand clients' current social support, its quality, and the way the client is (or is not) using their available support. Once the client has placed the names of their interpersonal supports on the inventory, the next step is for the clinician to explore each of the important relationships in depth. This exercise is designed to practice this skill. Questions that the clinician can ask while cocreating the inventory gather information about the quality of each of the client's relationships, including the interpersonal dynamics, accessibility of support, and the specific interpersonal difficulties that may be contributing or maintaining the presenting distress. The goal is to ask questions in a way that allows the client to describe their current relationships in detail.

In this exercise, you will practice asking questions about one of the client's relationships that they have noted on the inventory. The same types of questions will be asked about all their relationships. Over the full session, the goal is to gather information about each of the relationships the client lists. This process is usually done in Session 2.

https://doi.org/10.1037/0000426-004

Deliberate Practice in Interpersonal Psychotherapy, by O. Belik, J. M. Schultz, S. Fairhurst, S. Stuart, A. Vaz, and T. Rousmaniere

A great way to begin the information-collecting phase of the inventory is to start by asking the client, "Among the people you have listed on the Circle, who would you like to introduce me to first?" This question is a great way to collaborate with the client, model good communication skills, and allow the client to start where they feel most comfortable. It is assumed in this exercise that you have already had the client list names on the Circle (see Exercise 1).

In IPT clinical practice, you can ask as many questions as you need to understand the interpersonal support, interpersonal dynamics, and the accessibility the client has to the people on the inventory. A list of additional questions and troubleshooting is presented in Appendix D.

Clinicians should manage the session carefully so there is sufficient time to talk about every relationship. As a rule of thumb, talking about each relationship for about 5 minutes will usually leave sufficient time to ask five or six questions about every individual listed. Of course it is fine to spend a bit more or less time on each person depending on the importance of the specific relationship, and sometimes the inventory may take several sessions to complete.

The therapist should improvise a response to each client statement following these skill criteria:

1. **Praise the client for beginning the Interpersonal Inventory.** It is important to enhance your client's self-efficacy and ability to recognize and appraise their own achievement. Positive reinforcement, delivered well, is also a great way to model good communication. In addition, praise is a critical component in continuously engaging the client in treatment. A typical way to do this is, "Thanks for listing your support people on the Circle diagram; it gives me a nice visual picture of what your support looks like."

2. **Ask the client one (or more) question(s) (listed in the following box) to explore the specific relationship in more detail.** Exploring different aspects of the relationships between the client and other people they have listed on the inventory helps assess the quality and quantity of their current support.

3. **Practice using different questions for each client prompt.** To develop competency and confidence in using the Interpersonal Inventory, it is important to practice with a rich variety of questions. To the best of your ability, try varying the questions used in Criterion 2 throughout this practice.

SKILL CRITERIA FOR EXERCISE 2

1. Praise the client for beginning the Interpersonal Inventory.
2. Ask the client one or more question(s) from the following list to explore the specific relationship in more detail:
   - What do you appreciate the most about your relationship with this particular person?
   - In what way do you feel supported by this person, and how do you support this person in return?
   - What aspects of the relationship with this person do you appreciate the most, and what aspects of the relationship would you want to change?
   - How does the relationship with this person make you feel?
   - How do you and this person typically let each other know that you need help or support?
3. Practice using different questions from the previous list for each client prompt.

Examples of Therapists Exploring Interpersonal Relationships

Example 1

CLIENT: [*excited*] As I look at the Circle diagram, I think my cousin Joe stands out as the most important person in my life.

THERAPIST: I agree—thanks for writing the names on the Circle so we can both see them. (Criterion 1) Let's talk more about your relationship with Joe. What do you appreciate the most about your relationship with him? (Criterion 2)

Example 2

CLIENT: [*tentative*] I think I am done putting down names on the Circle diagram. I can start by talking about my mother.

THERAPIST: Good job getting this part of the inventory done. (Criterion 1) Since you want to start there, let's talk more about your relationship with your mother. What aspects of that relationship do you appreciate the most, and what aspects would you want to change? (Criterion 2)

Example 3

CLIENT: [*sad*] As you can see I don't have a lot of people in my Circle. I guess we can start with my sister if you want.

THERAPIST: Thank you for finishing this part, it helps me better understand your current support and why you may be having difficulty now. (Criterion 1) Let's stay with your idea to talk about your sister first. How do you and your sister support each other? (Criterion 2)

INSTRUCTIONS FOR EXERCISE 2

Step 1: Role-Play and Feedback

- The client says the first beginner client statement. The therapist **improvises** a response based on the skill criteria.
- The trainer (or, if not available, the client) provides **brief** feedback based on the skill criteria.
- The client then repeats the same statement, and the therapist again improvises a response. The trainer (or client) again provides brief feedback.

Step 2: Repeat

- Repeat Step 1 for all the statements **in the current difficulty level** (beginner, intermediate, or advanced).

Step 3: Assess and Adjust Difficulty

- The therapist completes the Deliberate Practice Reaction Form (see Appendix A) and decides whether to make the exercise easier or harder or to repeat the same difficulty level.

Step 4: Repeat for Approximately 15 Minutes

- Repeat Steps 1 to 3 for at least 15 minutes.
- The trainees then switch therapist and client roles and start over.

Now it's your turn! Follow Steps 1 and 2 from the instructions.

Remember: The goal of the role-play is for trainees to practice improvising responses to the client statements in a manner that (a) uses the skill criteria and (b) feels authentic for the trainee. **Example therapist responses for each client statement are provided at the end of this exercise. Trainees should attempt to improvise their own responses before reading the example responses.**

BEGINNER-LEVEL CLIENT STATEMENTS FOR EXERCISE 2
Beginner Client Statement 1
[Excited] OK, I am all done with the names! Can we start with my wife? She's the most important person for me.
Beginner Client Statement 2
[Engaged] I am all done putting down names. I can start by talking about my relationship with my brother.
Beginner Client Statement 3
[Proud] OK, I think I got everyone on the Circle! Maybe I can start with my sister . . .
Beginner Client Statement 4
[Hopeful] This was harder than I thought, but I am finished with the Circle. I picked my best friend to start with.
Beginner Client Statement 5
[Confident] This was interesting. I finished the Circle, and I think I got everyone I wanted in it! I want to talk about my neighbor first.

Assess and adjust the difficulty before moving to the next difficulty level (see Step 3 in the exercise instructions).

INTERMEDIATE-LEVEL CLIENT STATEMENTS FOR EXERCISE 2
Intermediate Client Statement 1
[Anticipation] OK, I'm all done. What do we do now? Can we start with my brother?
Intermediate Client Statement 2
[Worried] Here. These are the people in my Circle. I'm not sure if I placed people in the right place. Maybe I can start by telling you about my coworker.
Intermediate Client Statement 3
[Sad] Well, I finished, but I really don't have that many people in my Circle. Is that OK? The easiest to talk about first would be my sister.
Intermediate Client Statement 4
[Hesitant] So, I'm not sure if I got everyone in my Circle. I'm worried I might have forgotten someone. I guess starting with my aunt Cecilia would be OK. . . .
Intermediate Client Statement 5
[Anxious] It's hard for me to finish this. . . . I don't want to miss anyone. Since you told me to, I put down 10 people. Can we start with my friend Andrew?

🛑 **Assess and adjust the difficulty before moving to the next difficulty level (see Step 3 in the exercise instructions).**

ADVANCED-LEVEL CLIENT STATEMENTS FOR EXERCISE 2
Advanced Client Statement 1
[Gloomy] I just don't know . . . I guess that's it for my Circle. You want to look at it and make sure I did it right? Should we start with my father?
Advanced Client Statement 2
[Disengaged] OK, whatever. Here it is, the Circle you wanted. I guess we can start with my brother.
Advanced Client Statement 3
[Annoyance] Ugh, I am so annoyed at this activity and some of my people. I've been having lots of fights with my friends lately and thought about leaving them off. Maybe we can talk about my closest friend, Julia.
Advanced Client Statement 4
[Frustration] This is so frustrating! It's so hard to get all the people sorted out! I can start with my cousin, I guess.
Advanced Client Statement 5
[Anger] I'm so angry that some of these people left me over the years! I used to have more friends, but now I've got only a few that have been loyal. I'm angry at my friend Lauren, I don't want to talk about her though.

🛑 **Assess and adjust the difficulty here (see Step 3 in the exercise instructions). If appropriate, follow the instructions to make the exercise even more challenging (see Appendix A).**

Example Therapist Responses: Exploring Interpersonal Relationships

Remember: Trainees should attempt to improvise their own responses before reading the example responses. **Do not read the following responses verbatim unless you are having trouble coming up with your own!**

EXAMPLE RESPONSES TO BEGINNER-LEVEL CLIENT STATEMENTS FOR EXERCISE 2
Example Response to Beginner Client Statement 1
Great job completing this part of the Inventory! (Criterion 1) Yes, let's start by talking more about your relationship with your wife. What do you appreciate the most about your relationship with her? (Criterion 2)
Example Response to Beginner Client Statement 2
Good job finishing this part of the Circle! (Criterion 1) Tell me more about the way you feel supported by your brother and how do you support him in return? (Criterion 2)
Example Response to Beginner Client Statement 3
Well done getting everyone you wanted to in the Circle. (Criterion 1) I'll follow your lead and we can start by talking about your sister. What aspects of the relationship with your brother do you appreciate the most and what aspects of the relationship would you want to change? (Criterion 2)
Example Response to Beginner Client Statement 4
Yes, good work with Interpersonal Inventory! (Criterion 1) How does your relationship with your best friend make you feel? (Criterion 2)
Example Response to Beginner Client Statement 5
I'm glad you've already found the work we are doing together interesting. (Criterion 1) How do you and your neighbor let each other know that you need some support or help? (Criterion 2)

EXAMPLE RESPONSES TO INTERMEDIATE-LEVEL CLIENT STATEMENTS FOR EXERCISE 2

Example Response to Intermediate Client Statement 1

Good work finishing this part of the Inventory. (Criterion 1) Sure, I'd like to get more detailed information about your brother. How does your relationship with him make you feel? (Criterion 2)

Example Response to Intermediate Client Statement 2

Thanks for completing this part of the Inventory. As I mentioned before, there are no right or wrong ways to do it—I'm interested in your perspective. (Criterion 1) Since you suggested it, let's start with talking about your coworker. How do you feel supported by them, and how do you support them in return? (Criterion 2)

Example Response to Intermediate Client Statement 3

You did well by placing people you do have on the Circle. There is no right or wrong way to do it, and no right or wrong number to have on the Circle. (Criterion 1) Starting to get more details with your sister sounds good. What parts of your relationship with your sister do you appreciate the most, and what parts do you wish you could change? (Criterion 2)

Example Response to Intermediate Client Statement 4

Good job completing the Circle. We can always add more people later if you forgot someone. (Criterion 1) For now, as you suggested, let's talk about your aunt Cecilia. How does your relationship with her make you feel? (Criterion 2)

Example Response to Intermediate Client Statement 5

Yes, thanks for doing this part of the inventory exercise. Well done—there are no right or wrong ways to do it. (Criterion 1) It looks like you have quite a few people who support you. To get more details, how do you and Andrew let each other know that you need some help and support from each other? (Criterion 2)

EXAMPLE RESPONSES TO ADVANCED-LEVEL CLIENT STATEMENTS FOR EXERCISE 2
Example Response to Advanced Client Statement 1
Looks great to me—as I mentioned, there are no right or wrong ways to do it. This picture helps me better understand what your relationships are like, so thanks. (Criterion 1) We can certainly start with your father. What do you appreciate the most about your relationship with him? (Criterion 2)
Example Response to Advanced Client Statement 2
Thanks for finishing that part of the Circle—I appreciate knowing more about your supports, which I think will be really helpful to work from as we continue in therapy. (Criterion 1) Could you tell me more about what your relationship with your brother is like? (Criterion 2)
Example Response to Advanced Client Statement 3
You've done a great job of illustrating your relationships on the Circle so I can understand them better. (Criterion 1) I understand you've been having some conflicts with your friends. Yes, maybe we can start with Julia. What parts of your relationship with her do you appreciate the most, and which parts would you want to change? (Criterion 2)
Example Response to Advanced Client Statement 4
Thanks for doing this even though it wasn't easy. I appreciate that—I think that pushing through to get difficult things done will help you throughout our work together. (Criterion 1) Since you wanted to start with your cousin, tell me more about what you appreciate the most about that relationship. (Criterion 2)
Example Response to Advanced Client Statement 5
The anger you mention is helpful because it gives me a general sense about what your relationships are like and how they have changed, so thanks for that. (Criterion 1) I'd like to get more details about all the relationships on your Circle diagram, so who would you like to start with? How does your relationship with that person make you feel? (Criterion 2)

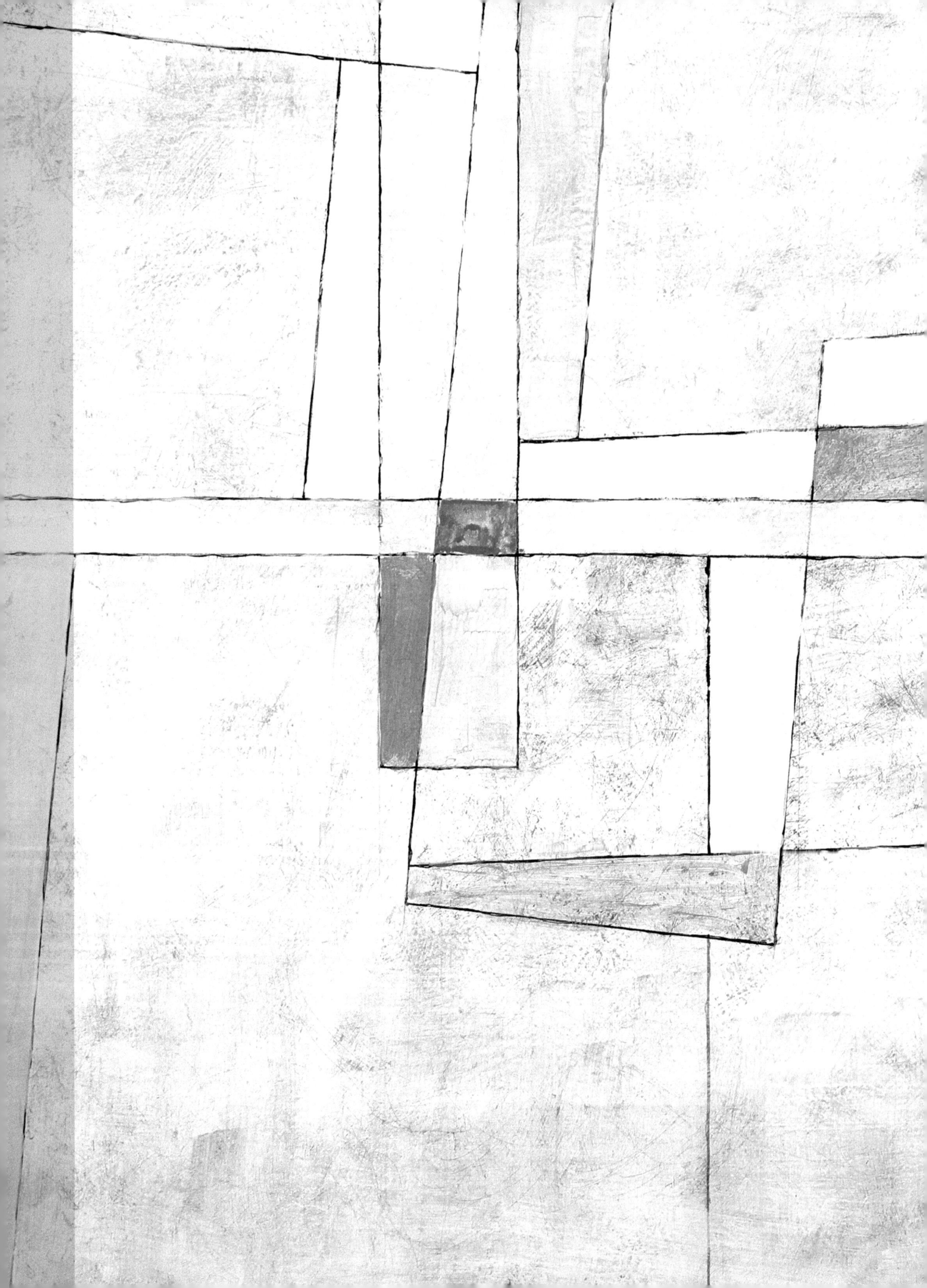

Clarifications

Preparations for Exercise 3

1. Read the instructions in Chapter 2.

2. Download the Deliberate Practice Reaction Form and the Deliberate Practice Diary Form at https://www.apa.org/pubs/books/deliberate-practice-interpersonal-psychotherapy (see the "Resources" tab; also available in Appendixes A and B, respectively).

Skill Description

Skill Difficulty Level: Beginner

Clarification is a skill frequently used in interpersonal psychotherapy (IPT) throughout the entire treatment. During the initial/assessment phase of the IPT, clarification is helpful for the purposes of information gathering and assisting the client to increase their awareness of the interpersonal dynamics and relational patterns. During the middle phase of the IPT, Clarification can be used to assist the client not only to understand but also to narrate their experiences and then explore options for change.

The therapist should improvise a response to each client statement following these skill criteria:

1. **Briefly and accurately summarize the client's statement.** It is critical for clinicians to make sure that they have an accurate understanding of their clients' experience to proceed with follow-up interventions. Summarizing a client's statements can assist the client in naming and organizing their emotional experiences and provide clarity about their situation. Lastly, providing clients with a summary of their statements can give them a unique feeling of feeling understood and felt by the clinician, which enhances the client–therapist working alliance.

https://doi.org/10.1037/0000426-005

Deliberate Practice in Interpersonal Psychotherapy, by O. Belik, J. M. Schultz, S. Fairhurst, S. Stuart, A. Vaz, and T. Rousmaniere

2. **Ask the client a question that helps them further describe their experience.** It is helpful to the client to be able to elaborate on their interpersonal experiences because these contribute to the client's mood and, ultimately, impact their functioning. By further describing their experience, clients gain awareness and insight into their interpersonal dynamics. When the client has clarity about their interpersonal situation, their whole situation starts to make sense. This can increase the client's commitment to change, motivation for treatment, and adherence for assignments between therapy sessions.

SKILL CRITERIA FOR EXERCISE 3

1. Briefly and accurately summarize the client's statement.
2. Ask the client a question that helps them further describe their experience.

Examples of Therapists Using Clarification

Example 1

CLIENT: [*sad*] I saw my girlfriend yesterday and we again got in a fight. . . . I wish I could do something about these fights that keep happening; it brings me down every single time.

THERAPIST: I hear how sad and tired you are from fighting with your girlfriend and I also hear you wanting to be able to do something about it so that you do not fight as often. (Criterion 1) What is it like for you when you keep fighting? (Criterion 2)

Example 2

CLIENT: [*confused*] I am not sure what happened last week at my volleyball game. I told my coach that I was tired and needed a break, but he ignored me and now I don't know how to communicate with him when it's too much for me. He usually listens, but this time I did not feel understood.

THERAPIST: Sounds like your coach is usually responsive when you communicate with him, but since you feel that you communicated well last week, but were ignored, you now worry if you will feel understood by your coach in the future. (Criterion 1) What was that experience like for you to not feel understood? (Criterion 2)

Example 3

CLIENT: [*excited*] Things are now OK with my best friend at school! We were playing handball and I just told her how she made me feel last night and she agreed that she was too focused on the game and did not know how I was feeling. I asked her not to talk to me this way again, and she agreed. I am so glad! I was able to talk to her!

THERAPIST: Sounds like you had a good conversation with your friend where you were able to express your feelings and to set expectations for future communications. Sounds like you feel positive and proud that you were able to talk to your friend in an open and honest way. (Criterion 1) What was that experience of being able to communicate your feelings felt like? (Criterion 2)

INSTRUCTIONS FOR EXERCISE 3

Step 1: Role-Play and Feedback

- The client says the first beginner client statement. The therapist **improvises** a response based on the skill criteria.
- The trainer (or, if not available, the client) provides **brief** feedback based on the skill criteria.
- The client then repeats the same statement, and the therapist again improvises a response. The trainer (or client) again provides brief feedback.

Step 2: Repeat

- Repeat Step 1 for all the statements **in the current difficulty level** (beginner, intermediate, or advanced).

Step 3: Assess and Adjust Difficulty

- The therapist completes the Deliberate Practice Reaction Form (see Appendix A) and decides whether to make the exercise easier or harder or to repeat the same difficulty level.

Step 4: Repeat for Approximately 15 Minutes

- Repeat Steps 1 to 3 for at least 15 minutes.
- The trainees then switch therapist and client roles and start over.

Now it's your turn! Follow Steps 1 and 2 from the exercise instructions.

Remember: The goal of the role-play is for trainees to practice improvising responses to the client statements in a manner that (a) uses the skill criteria and (b) feels authentic for the trainee. **Example therapist responses for each client statement are provided at the end of this exercise. Trainees should attempt to improvise their own responses before reading the example responses.**

BEGINNER-LEVEL CLIENT STATEMENTS FOR EXERCISE 3
Beginner Client Statement 1
[Sad] I had a conversation with my friend about our upcoming trip and I think I hurt her feelings. I feel so sad that I hurt her feelings—she's my friend! I don't know what to do next.
Beginner Client Statement 2
[Excited] I had such a great time with my family last night! I don't remember the last time we all got along so well. It gives me hope for our future gatherings!
Beginner Client Statement 3
[Worried] I'm nervous about the conversation that I want to have with my mother. I want to tell her that I am no longer interested in participating in dance lessons. This has been an important decision that I've made for myself.
Beginner Client Statement 4
[Hesitant] I really don't know if I want to be with my boyfriend. I care for him, but I am not sure if I still love him. I wish I could understand my own feelings better!
Beginner Client Statement 5
[Happy] I am so very excited! My sister decided to come visit me and we have not seen each other in about 3 years!

 Assess and adjust the difficulty before moving to the next difficulty level (see Step 3 in the exercise instructions).

INTERMEDIATE-LEVEL CLIENT STATEMENTS FOR EXERCISE 3
Intermediate Client Statement 1
[Upset] I can't believe I had such a terrible conversation with my brother! I am so upset at how he made me feel and now I have no idea what to do about it.
Intermediate Client Statement 2
[Anxious] So, I finally made a decision to talk to my boss, but now I am worried about it. I want to make sure I communicate clearly, and I worry I might not be direct enough.
Intermediate Client Statement 3
[Unsure] How do I repair the fight with my friend? I am not sure what is the best way to approach her.
Intermediate Client Statement 4
[Angry] I am so angry at my neighbors! They have been blasting the music until 11 p.m. for the last three nights! It's so late, and I can't fall asleep for a while after they stop their music. I really need to talk to them about it, but I just don't know how to have that conversation.
Intermediate Client Statement 5
[Worry] I worry about my upcoming performance review. I have not been happy with my own performance because I was traveling for my family emergency so much.

 Assess and adjust the difficulty before moving to the next difficulty level (see Step 3 in the exercise instructions).

ADVANCED-LEVEL CLIENT STATEMENTS FOR EXERCISE 3
Advanced Client Statement 1
[Disappointed] This situation at work feels more complicated than I thought it would. I am not sure what to do about my work situation. I'm disappointed in my boss who I used to admire.
Advanced Client Statement 2
[Sad] I'm so sad, I miss my mom! I wish she was still alive and could spend some time with my kids and they could feel how loving she was.
Advanced Client Statement 3
[Confused] I'm so torn about my dad. As you know, he has never been present in my life but all of a sudden he wants to be involved and have input into my life. I think I'm happy and sad all at the same time, not sure what to feel.
Advanced Client Statement 4
[Ambivalent] I'm so proud that I got an offer from the job I interviewed for last week! But now I feel sad having to leave my current work and the friends that I made here. I feel like I now have mixed feelings about starting a new job.
Advanced Client Statement 5
[Anxious] It has been really difficult for me to think about "coming out" to my family. It is really important to be who I truly am when I am with my family. I keep thinking, what if they reject me? What am I going to do if they don't want me to be a part of the family anymore?

> 🛑 **Assess and adjust the difficulty here (see Step 3 in the exercise instructions). If appropriate, follow the instructions to make the exercise even more challenging (see Appendix A).**

Example Therapist Responses: Clarifications

Remember: Trainees should attempt to improvise their own responses before reading the example responses. **Do not read the following responses verbatim unless you are having trouble coming up with your own responses!**

EXAMPLE RESPONSES TO BEGINNER-LEVEL CLIENT STATEMENTS FOR EXERCISE 3
Example Response to Beginner Client Statement 1
It sounds like you feel sad for hurting your friend's feelings and now you are wondering what to do next. (Criterion 1) What was it like for you to realize you hurt her feelings? (Criterion 2)
Example Response to Beginner Client Statement 2
I can see and feel happiness in your voice! I am so glad you had a wonderful time with your family, you have been hoping the gathering would go well. (Criterion 1) What was it like for you to enjoy your family time with everyone? (Criterion 2)
Example Response to Beginner Client Statement 3
Sounds like the conversation with your mother is important to you and you worry about how she will respond to your decision. (Criterion 1) What was that process like for you to make a decision not to participate in dance lessons anymore? (Criterion 2)
Example Response to Beginner Client Statement 4
Sounds like you are unsure about your feelings and it's unclear to you if you want to stay in a relationship with your boyfriend. (Criterion 1) Can you tell me more about the complexity of your feelings toward your boyfriend? (Criterion 2)
Example Response to Beginner Client Statement 5
I can see and feel your excitement about reconnecting with your sister! (Criterion 1) What does it feel like to know you are about to see your sister and spend some time with her, just the two of you? (Criterion 2)

EXAMPLE RESPONSES TO INTERMEDIATE-LEVEL CLIENT STATEMENTS FOR EXERCISE 3
Example Response to Intermediate Client Statement 1
Sounds like a conversation with your brother left you feeling upset and now you are not sure what to do next. (Criterion 1) Can you talk a bit about the conversation with your brother that left you feeling so upset? (Criterion 2)
Example Response to Intermediate Client Statement 2
I hear you say a couple of things here: You made a decision to talk to your boss, and you worry if you can communicate clearly during that conversation. (Criterion 1) Can you speak about your intention to talk to your boss and what exactly you would like to say? (Criterion 2)
Example Response to Intermediate Client Statement 3
Sounds like there was a fight between you and your friend and you would like to repair the relationship. I also hear that you are not quite sure how to go about the repair. (Criterion 1) Can you talk about the fight that you both had? Maybe that will help us generate some options for repair. (Criterion 2)
Example Response to Intermediate Client Statement 4
I am hearing a couple of things: First, your neighbor's playing music until 11 p.m. is really impacting your ability to sleep and you would like to have a conversation with them. I am also hearing you are not sure how to approach that conversation. (Criterion 1) Can you tell me more about your experience and what you would like to tell them? (Criterion 2)
Example Response to Intermediate Client Statement 5
Let me see if I understand your situation. You have been away from your job taking care of your family needs and you are worried about the upcoming performance evaluation at work as you think that your being away affected your performance. (Criterion 1) Can you talk a bit more about the impact that you think you being away from work had on your performance? (Criterion 2)

EXAMPLE RESPONSES TO ADVANCED-LEVEL CLIENT STATEMENTS FOR EXERCISE 3

Example Response to Advanced Client Statement 1

I am hearing a couple of things: One, I hear you are disappointed in your boss and feel the loss of respect for them. I am also hearing that there is a complicated situation at work that you are unsure how to handle. (Criterion 1) Can you tell me more about your current experience at work? (Criterion 2)

Example Response to Advanced Client Statement 2

It saddens you that your kids cannot experience your mom and feel loved by her. You miss her being a part of everyone's life. (Criterion 1) What would it be like to have your mom around? (Criterion 2)

Example Response to Advanced Client Statement 3

Let me summarize what I think I am hearing. On one hand, you are glad your dad is back in your life; at the same time, you feel sad knowing that he has not been present until now. (Criterion 1) What does it feel like having your dad back in your life while knowing he has not been around? (Criterion 2)

Example Response to Advanced Client Statement 4

I hear your ambivalence about moving forward with your new job and leaving behind your current work. On one hand, you are proud of yourself for getting the job you wanted; on the other, you feel sad about saying goodbye to friends at your current job. (Criterion 1) What does it feel like to have such complicated feelings about your current job situation? (Criterion 2)

Example Response to Advanced Client Statement 5

I hear how imperative it is for you to be who you truly are with your family. On one hand, it is important for you to come out to them; on the other, you worry about their reaction and whether they will accept you for who you are. (Criterion 1) What is it like for you to be in this space of wanting to honor who you are while worrying about your family's reaction? (Criterion 2)

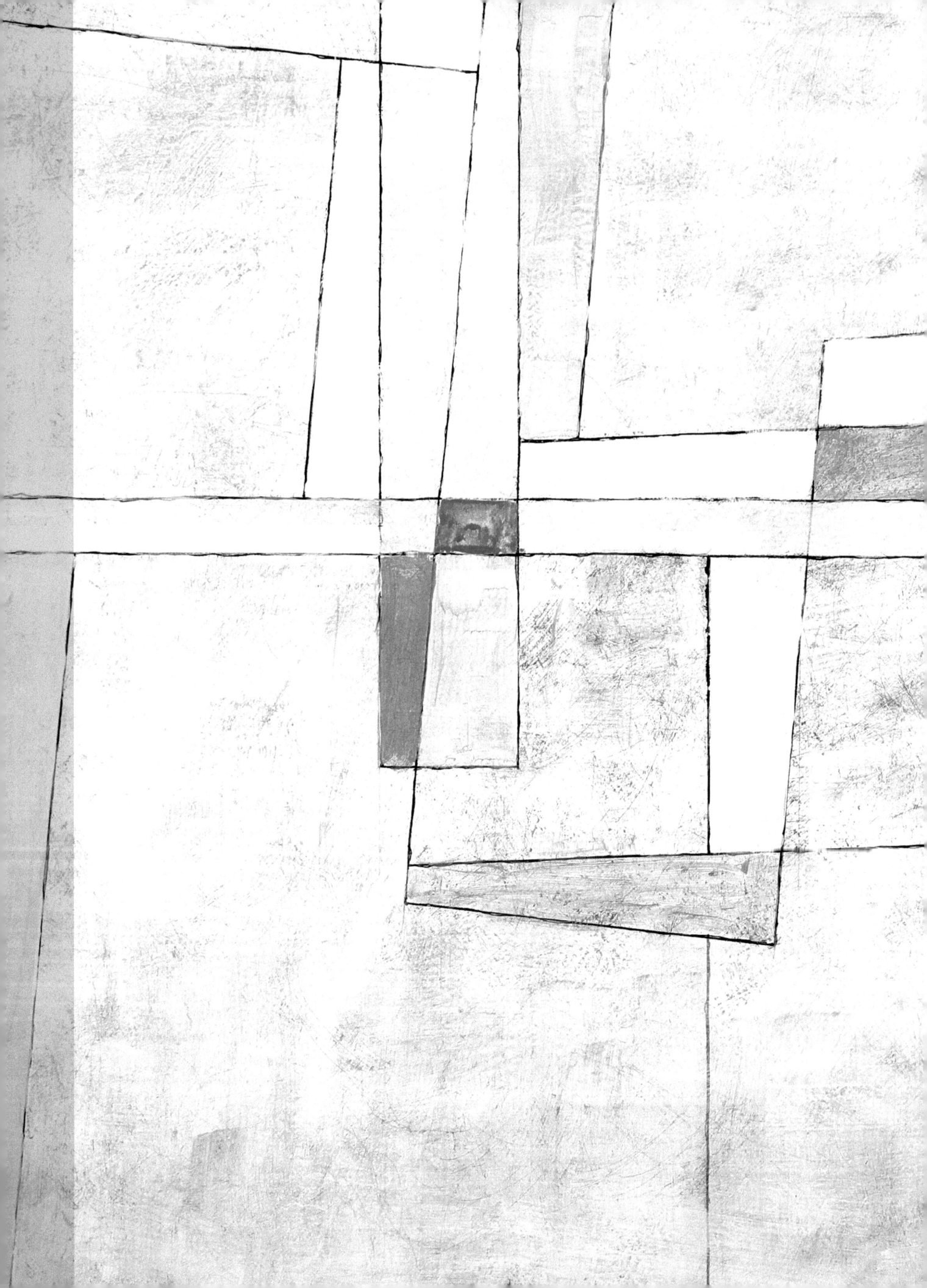

Interpersonal Framing
of Distress

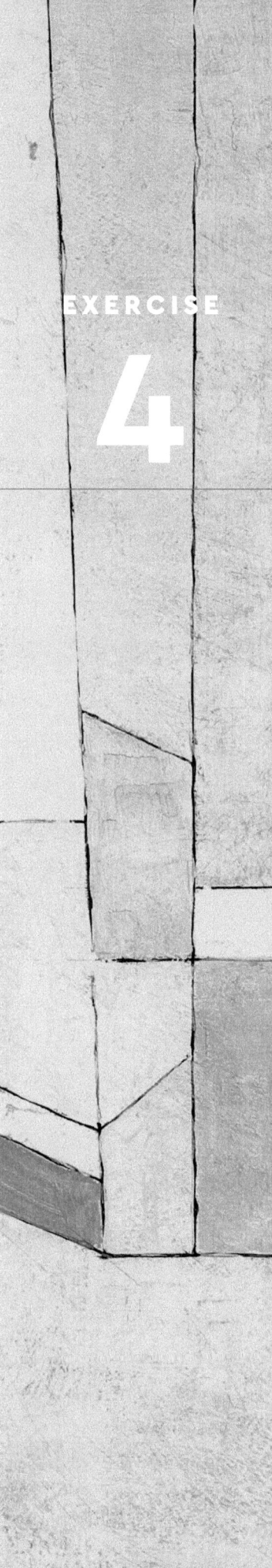

Preparations for Exercise 4

1. Read the instructions in Chapter 2.

2. Download the Deliberate Practice Reaction Form and the Deliberate Practice Diary Form at https://www.apa.org/pubs/books/deliberate-practice-interpersonal-psychotherapy (see the "Resources" tab; also available in Appendixes A and B, respectively).

Skill Description

Skill Difficulty Level: Intermediate

Conceptualizing *why* distress is happening is essential in all psychotherapeutic models. That conceptualization is not only important for the therapist; it is also critical for the client to understand how they came to be distressed and what is perpetuating it. Given the highly collaborative nature of interpersonal psychotherapy (IPT), creating and maintaining a shared understanding between the client and therapist about what is contributing to the distress is an important element of therapy. That shared understanding will then lead to a clear focus for treatment.

This is done in IPT by developing an interpersonal frame for the client's distress. This interpersonal frame focuses IPT treatment on improving relationships and increasing social support as the mechanisms for change. The interpersonal framing of distress skill is especially important early in IPT but may be used throughout therapy as issues arise to maintain and sharpen focus on relational themes.

Clients present with a range of symptoms and problems that can be described in many different ways. Using the interpersonal framing of distress skill, the therapist identifies and summarizes the interpersonal factors contributing to distress to help clients understand and organize what is happening in their social network and on which relationships

https://doi.org/10.1037/0000426-006

Deliberate Practice in Interpersonal Psychotherapy, by O. Belik, J. M. Schultz, S. Fairhurst, S. Stuart, A. Vaz, and T. Rousmaniere

therapy should focus. The *relational frame* conceptualization in IPT is the concept that the client's experience of distress affects those around them and that the people supporting (or failing to support) the client impact the client's experiences of distress. These interpersonal factors might include relational conflict or disconnection, difficult life transitions, loss of relationship, lack of social support, and feeling unheard or misunderstood by others.

Importantly, using this skill, the therapist is not providing an "interpretation" to the client or providing a definitive description about what is happening and why the client is in distress. Instead, as described and practiced in Exercise 3, the therapist uses clarification skills to invite the client to summarize the interpersonal factors that are likely to be at play and then invites the client to respond. This collaborative approach allows space for the client(s) to offer their perspectives, which serves to develop and strengthen a *shared understanding* of distress. Not only is the conceptualization of distress likely to be more accurate, but this approach also strengthens the therapeutic alliance.

The therapist should improvise a response to each client statement following these skill criteria:

1. **Reflect/validate the client's distress.** A strong therapeutic alliance is critical to the success of any treatment, including IPT. The alliance is facilitated by the clinician communicating empathy and working to understand the client. The interpersonal framing of distress skill begins with the clinician briefly reflecting or validating the client's distress to communicate empathy and that they are working to understand the client better. For example, the therapist might say, "It sounds like you have been through a lot. Based on what you've described, I think I understand more about what you are going through and what we can do to help you."

2. **Connect the client's distress with interpersonal issues they are experiencing.** IPT focuses on the interpersonal factors in the client's life that are creating and/or maintaining psychological distress. Focusing on these interpersonal factors in treatment is one of the mechanisms of change in IPT. To build a shared understanding of the distress between therapist and client, it is critical for IPT trainees to learn to "translate" the client's concerns by homing in on the explicit or implicit interpersonal nature of these concerns. A typical intervention is: "Based on what you have described so far, it sounds like a lot of the distress you are experiencing is connected to the loss of your grandfather. Losses, particularly those of people close to us, are really difficult."

3. **Check to determine if this potential connection makes sense to the client.** IPT is a highly collaborative treatment built on a strong therapeutic alliance and shared understanding of the problem(s). It is critical for therapists to use and model good communication skills in service of deepening the alliance and client investment in treatment, especially when offering explanations using the interpersonal framing of distress. After offering an interpersonal connection for the client's distress, the clinician should offer the opportunity and space for the client to respond to, expand on, and/or correct the clinician's assessment. For example, the therapist might say, "What do you think of the connection I am thinking about regarding your depression and your grandfather's death? Does that make sense to you? How would you add to it?"

SKILL CRITERIA FOR EXERCISE 4
1. Reflect and validate the client's distress.
2. Connect the client's distress with interpersonal issues they are experiencing.
3. Check to determine if this potential connection makes sense to the client.

Examples of Therapists Using Interpersonal Framing of Distress

Note: All client statements in this particular exercise take place in the initial/assessment phase of IPT after the client has completed the Interpersonal Inventory. They can later be used to generate the IPT Summary goals with the client at the end of the initial/assessment phase. Of course, this skill can also be used throughout treatment as concerns are presented and evolve.

Example 1

CLIENT: [*sad*] I don't know what to do. I keep thinking about my ex-wife. I'm super alone, I can't sleep right, and I don't even feel like eating any more.

THERAPIST: How difficult it must be for you to not be able to sleep or eat and to feel so alone. (Criterion 1) It sounds to me like a lot of that is connected to the loss of your relationship with your ex-partner, which is really impacting your daily functioning. (Criterion 2) How does that strike you? (Criterion 3)

Example 2

CLIENT: [*angry*] I can't believe my dad is dead. This isn't fair! We were supposed to have so much more time together. I can't stop thinking about how unfair his death is and about how I'll never see him again.

THERAPIST: It's completely understandable that you are feeling so angry and sad that you can't stop thinking about him. Loss is hard for everyone. (Criterion 1) It seems to me like your dad's death and missing him has almost certainly led to you feeling this way. (Criterion 2) Am I understanding that well? (Criterion 3)

Example 3

CLIENT: [*anxious*] I'm failing in this class I'm taking, and I'm feeling really nervous about approaching my teacher for help. I don't know who else to turn to.

THERAPIST: I can see how anxious you're feeling, and why that is likely to be the case. (Criterion 1) It seems to me that the lack of support for your academic work is really affecting how you're doing in class and how you're feeling overall. (Criterion 2) Am I on track in connecting the lack of support you are describing with how anxious you're feeling? (Criterion 3)

INSTRUCTIONS FOR EXERCISE 4

Step 1: Role-Play and Feedback

- The client says the first beginner client statement. The therapist **improvises** a response based on the skill criteria.
- The trainer (or, if not available, the client) provides **brief** feedback based on the skill criteria.
- The client then repeats the same statement, and the therapist again improvises a response. The trainer (or client) again provides brief feedback.

Step 2: Repeat

- Repeat Step 1 for all the statements **in the current difficulty level** (beginner, intermediate, or advanced).

Step 3: Assess and Adjust Difficulty

- The therapist completes the Deliberate Practice Reaction Form (see Appendix A) and decides whether to make the exercise easier or harder or to repeat the same difficulty level.

Step 4: Repeat for Approximately 15 Minutes

- Repeat Steps 1 to 3 for at least 15 minutes.
- The trainees then switch therapist and client roles and start over.

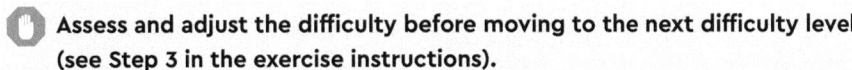

Now it's your turn! Follow Steps 1 and 2 from the instructions.

Remember: The goal of the role-play is for trainees to practice improvising responses to the client statements in a manner that (a) uses the skill criteria and (b) feels authentic for the trainee. **Example therapist responses for each client statement are provided at the end of this exercise. Trainees should attempt to improvise their own responses before reading the example responses.**

BEGINNER-LEVEL CLIENT STATEMENTS FOR EXERCISE 4
Beginner Client Statement 1
[Frustrated] All we do anymore is argue. All the time. About money, about the kids, about the house, about everything. It just never stops, and I don't know much more I can take.
Beginner Client Statement 2
[Sad] I miss home. I miss my friends. I miss my teacher. I miss my dog. Maybe college just isn't for me.
Beginner Client Statement 3
[Resigned] I don't know what to do with my family anymore. When we're together, I can't stop thinking about who they voted for and how different our values are now. So I try to avoid seeing them and talking to them, but I feel like there's a big hole in my life.
Beginner Client Statement 4
[Frustrated] I feel like no one at work takes me seriously. They talk over me in meetings and never really listen to what I have to say. I wish I could just leave, but I have to make a living somehow and I need this job.
Beginner Client Statement 5
[Annoyed] My parents just don't get it. They don't understand what it is like to grow up here in the States. They think I should just study all the time and not have a life. I know they care about me, but they made me come with them and now they're making things worse.

Assess and adjust the difficulty before moving to the next difficulty level (see Step 3 in the exercise instructions).

INTERMEDIATE-LEVEL CLIENT STATEMENTS FOR EXERCISE 4
Intermediate Client Statement 1
[Hopeless] How can I ever go on after this? Everyone acts like things are normal, but I'll never get over this miscarriage. I lost our baby, and it is my fault.
Intermediate Client Statement 2
[Sad] It was a terrible weekend. I couldn't get out of bed, so I just looked out the window watching all the people laughing, walking, and sitting at the cafe across the street from my apartment.
Intermediate Client Statement 3
[Overwhelmed] Since my dad's dementia diagnosis, I feel like I can't catch a break. I spend all day, every day arguing with the care facility and insurance company. Yesterday, I spent 3 hours at the bank trying to figure out his accounts. I try to spend all the time I can with him, but it just isn't the same, and I feel like the rest of my life is falling apart.
Intermediate Client Statement 4
[Apathetic] I know I should be happy to have a healthy baby. People keep telling me how cute he is, but all I can think about is how I have to breastfeed again in 30 minutes and battle him to go to sleep every time. I look at myself in the mirror, and I don't even know who I am anymore. No one understands.
Intermediate Client Statement 5
[Angry] How could she have an affair and do this to me? All I can think about is what she did. I'm in the grocery store, and I think about them cooking dinner. I'm in the school pick up line, and I wonder what she said to her about me. I see her with our kids, and I just want to scream. I can't stop thinking about it.

✋ **Assess and adjust the difficulty before moving to the next difficulty level (see Step 3 in the exercise instructions).**

ADVANCED-LEVEL CLIENT STATEMENTS FOR EXERCISE 4
Advanced Client Statement 1
[Dejected] I just can't do this job anymore. It is sucking the life out of me.
Advanced Client Statement 2
[Anxious] I can't stop thinking about my mom's cancer diagnosis. I'm sure she's going to die.
Advanced Client Statement 3
[Hopeless] How could this have happened? . . . He was my best friend. I never thought he could rape me. And I can't tell our friends because they won't believe me, and I bet some of them will even blame me.
Advanced Client Statement 4
[Enraged] How dare my stepdad think he can tell me what to do! He's not my real dad and he never will be.
Advanced Client Statement 5
[Hopeless] Things are never going to get better until my parents let me leave this homophobic school full of bullies.

🛑 **Assess and adjust the difficulty here (see Step 3 in the exercise instructions). If appropriate, follow the instructions to make the exercise even more challenging (see Appendix A).**

Example Therapist Responses: Interpersonal Framing of Distress

Remember: Trainees should attempt to improvise their own responses before reading the example responses. **Do not read the following responses verbatim unless you are having trouble coming up with your own!**

EXAMPLE RESPONSES TO BEGINNER-LEVEL CLIENT STATEMENTS FOR EXERCISE 4
Example Response to Beginner Client Statement 1
I hear you saying you are close to your limit of frustration (Criterion 1) and that it is this conflict with your partner that is causing the distress for you. (Criterion 2) Am I understanding that correctly? (Criterion 3)
Example Response to Beginner Client Statement 2
This transition to college is enormous for you, and it's changed so many of your relationships. (Criterion 1) It makes sense to me that these changes in your support system leave you feeling overwhelmed by it all. (Criterion 2) How does that fit with how you understand what is happening? (Criterion 3)
Example Response to Beginner Client Statement 3
It seems like you are feeling really disconnected from your family right now, (Criterion 1) and that disconnection from them is leading you to feel distressed. (Criterion 2) Am I understanding that correctly? (Criterion 3)
Example Response to Beginner Client Statement 4
It sounds like you aren't feeling heard or supported in your relationships with your coworkers (Criterion 1) and that this is likely leading to the frustration you are feeling. (Criterion 2) What do you think about that way of explaining what is happening? (Criterion 3)
Example Response to Beginner Client Statement 5
I can hear your deep frustration—that actually helps me better understand what this is like for you. (Criterion 1) It seems like your relationship with your parents and not feeling understood by them is a key factor in understanding the distress you are describing. (Criterion 2) Does that make sense to you? (Criterion 3)

EXAMPLE RESPONSES TO INTERMEDIATE-LEVEL CLIENT STATEMENTS FOR EXERCISE 4

Example Response to Intermediate Client Statement 1

I'm so sorry for your loss. Losing your baby and feeling like no one understands is unbelievably difficult, (Criterion 1) and it makes sense that both this loss and the disconnection you're feeling from others are creating pain for you. (Criterion 2) Am I capturing what is happening to you well? (Criterion 3)

Example Response to Intermediate Client Statement 2

It sounds like you are really feeling lonely and disconnected from others right now, (Criterion 1) and it seems like this is really contributing to your depression and distress. (Criterion 2) How does that fit with how you understand things? (Criterion 3)

Example Response to Intermediate Client Statement 3

It's got to be incredibly difficult to be juggling so many things right now, especially with your dad's illness. (Criterion 1) It seems like feeling a lack of support in managing all the caregiving tasks on top of coping with the changing relationship with your father is what is leading to you feeling like this. (Criterion 2) How does that fit with your understanding of what is happening? (Criterion 3)

Example Response to Intermediate Client Statement 4

Having a baby has changed so many things about your life. (Criterion 1) It seems like there is a lack of support in your life—people don't understand how difficult this is for you and how it has impacted everything about your life, and this is contributing to how you've been feeling. (Criterion 2) What do you think about that? (Criterion 3)

Example Response to Intermediate Client Statement 5

I'm so sorry. You experienced a major betrayal in your relationship with your partner—no wonder you're struggling right now. (Criterion 1) It makes sense to me that the rupture in your relationship is leading you to the distress you feel. (Criterion 2) How does that fit with your understanding of why you are feeling the way you do? (Criterion 3)

EXAMPLE RESPONSES TO ADVANCED-LEVEL CLIENT STATEMENTS FOR EXERCISE 4
Example Response to Advanced Client Statement 1
It sounds like the intensity of your work has left you disconnected from your support system, (Criterion 1) and this disconnection is leading to you feeling the way you do right now. (Criterion 2) Did I capture that accurately? (Criterion 3)
Example Response to Advanced Client Statement 2
What you're experiencing would be incredibly difficult for anyone. (Criterion 1) Am I understanding correctly that your concern about your mom's health, your relationship with your mom, and the need for more support as you navigate this diagnosis is leading you to feel distressed? (Criteria 2 and 3)
Example Response to Advanced Client Statement 3
I'm so sorry that happened to you. It wasn't your fault. (Criterion 1) I can see how the rape has been devastating, not to mention how isolated and unsupported you have felt since it happened. The feeling of isolation and lack of support have caused you to experience even more pain. (Criterion 2) Am I understanding correctly what that is like for you? (Criterion 3)
Example Response to Advanced Client Statement 4
It sounds really difficult to navigate things with your stepdad right now. (Criterion 1) It makes sense that the conflict with him, and trying to navigate your relationship with him is causing so much pain for you right now. (Criterion 2) How does that fit with how you understand why you've been feeling the way you've been feeling? (Criterion 3)
Example Response to Advanced Client Statement 5
I'm very sorry for all that you've been through at your school and the impact it has had on you. (Criterion 1) I can see how the bullying, the isolation, and your feeling that your parents don't understand how difficult it is for you is contributing to the distress you are feeling. (Criterion 2) How does that fit with how you see things? (Criterion 3)

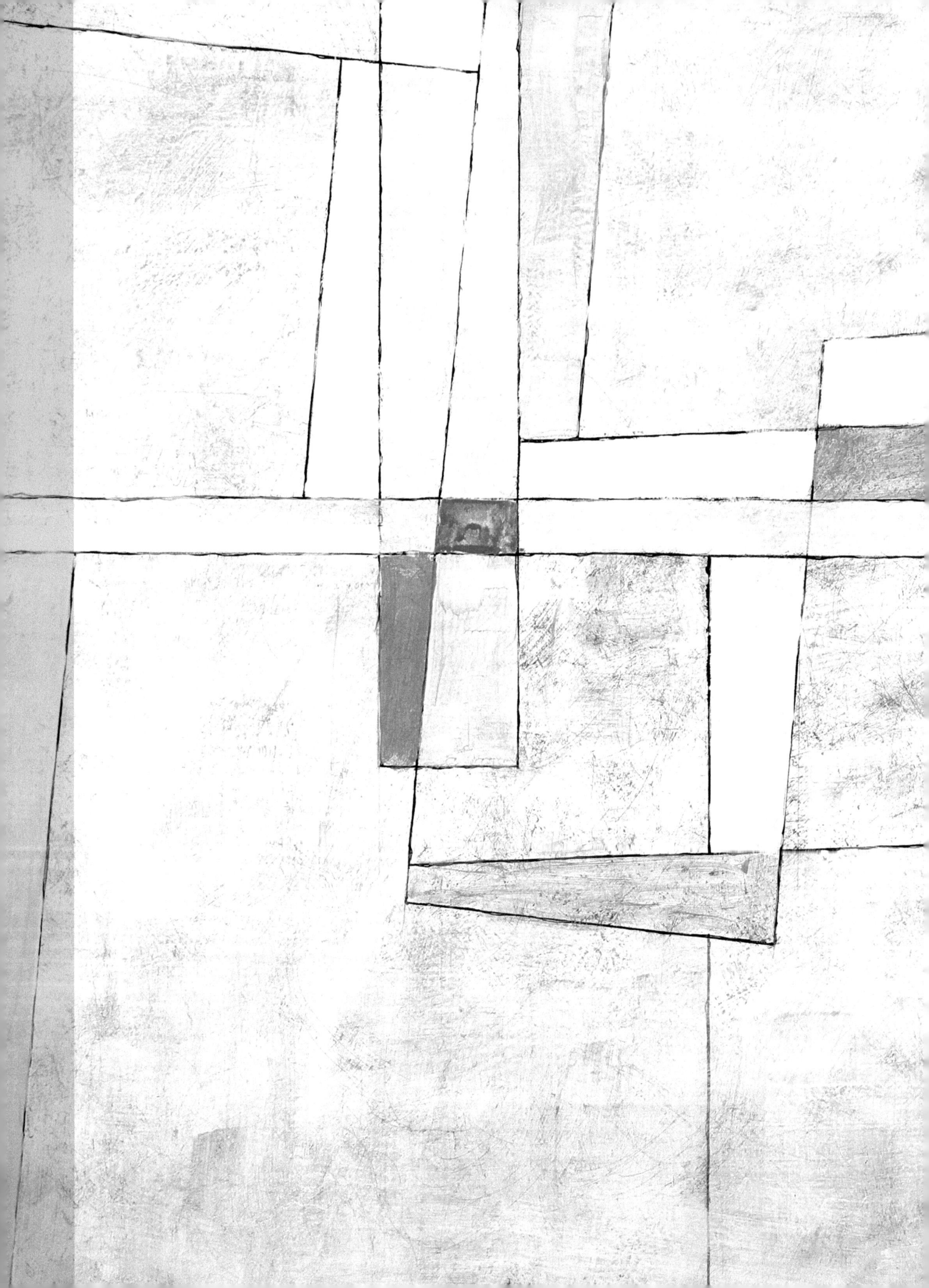

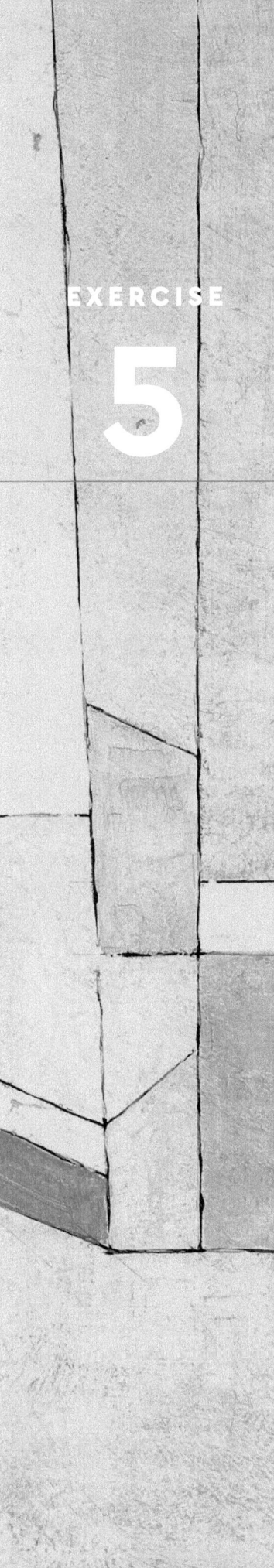

Helping the Client to Describe Their Distress and Need for Support

Preparations for Exercise 5

1. Read the instructions in Chapter 2.

2. Download the Deliberate Practice Reaction Form and the Deliberate Practice Diary Form at https://www.apa.org/pubs/books/deliberate-practice-interpersonal-psychotherapy (see the "Resources" tab; also available in Appendixes A and B, respectively).

Skill Description

Skill Difficulty Level: Intermediate

Understanding our emotions and interpersonal needs is complex, yet it is important to communicate them to ask for and receive the support that we need. Crises, and the interpersonal distress they cause, often make it even more difficult for clients to know what they need, much less how to ask for it well. The result is often that clients either do not ask for support or ask for it in unproductive ways that make it difficult for others to respond well, and their distress increases further.

Helping the client to describe their distress and need for support is a skill that seeks to build the client's ability to ask graciously for the *specific* support that would be helpful. *Graciousness* in this context refers to a way of asking pleasantly, directly, and with gratitude for the help that is provided. In a very simple sense, it is teaching the patient to use words such as "please" and "thank you" to ask for and express appreciation for the support that others provide. Communicating in this way will increase the likelihood that support will be provided and that it will be provided again in the future if needed.

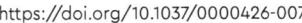

https://doi.org/10.1037/0000426-007

Deliberate Practice in Interpersonal Psychotherapy, by O. Belik, J. M. Schultz, S. Fairhurst, S. Stuart, A. Vaz, and T. Rousmaniere

This skill serves two primary purposes in interpersonal psychotherapy. First, it helps clients recognize and acknowledge both the practical and emotional needs in their relationships. Some clients may already be aware of this need, while identifying an emotional need may be a new insight for others. Second, this skill prompts clients to define what kind of *specific* help is needed and what it would look like in their relationships with others. Describing these needs in clear and specific ways lays the groundwork for clients to be able to ask for more clearly in ways that others in their Interpersonal Circle can understand and respond to.

This skill builds on two previous skills that have already been described and practiced. First, the Interpersonal Inventory must be developed (Exercise 1) because it is from some of the individuals on the Circle that the patient will eventually be communicating their desire for support. Second, understanding the quality of the relationships on the Circle (Exercises 2 and 4) will allow the therapist and client to choose which of the individuals on the client's Circle will be most likely to respond positively and which individuals are not likely to be able to provide help even if asked to do so in an appropriate way.

Helping the client to describe their distress and need for support also uses clarification techniques (Exercise 3) to help the client better understand and describe their needs. Action-oriented techniques such as *mobilizing social support* and *motivating interpersonal action* (covered in later exercises) may follow to help clients implement the insight they have gained and to mobilize or expand their support network.

The therapist should improvise a response to each client statement following these skill criteria:

1. **Summarize the emotional need of the client.** First, the clinician works gently to summarize or clarify the needs the client is describing. Clarifying the interpersonal emotional needs for support both validates the client's emotional experience and models ways in which the client can subsequently express it to others. The clinician should be intentional in framing the client's needs within an interpersonal context, meaning it is a need for support that can be met by another person (even if it isn't yet clear who that other person might be). A typical intervention is "It sounds like you're really struggling with a sense of isolation. Based on what you've described, I can't help but think that having someone simply be with you, whether to do an activity together or simply talk, would be really helpful."

2. **Prompt the client to explain specifically what the fulfillment of that need would look like in their relationships.** After the need is understood, the clinician uses opening questions or statements to invite the client to describe what it would look for that need to be met. This step deepens the client's understanding of the need and how they might ask for it to be met. To do this, clients may be invited to describe what meeting the interpersonal emotional need could look like and reflect on how it has been met in the past. Clearly defining what it looks like to have the need met will be extremely helpful when the client eventually asks their support network to meet it. A typical intervention is "How would you describe what you need in specific terms? How could you ask one of the people in your Circle for that kind of support?"

SKILL CRITERIA FOR EXERCISE 5

1. Summarize the emotional need of the client.
2. Prompt the client to explain specifically what the fulfillment of that need would look like in their relationships.

Examples of Therapists Helping the Client to Describe Their Distress and Need for Support

Example 1

CLIENT: [*dejected*] I don't feel like I matter in my relationship with my husband.

THERAPIST: Understandably—everyone wants to feel like a priority to their partner. (Criterion 1) What would need to happen for you to feel like you are a priority? (Criterion 2)

Example 2

CLIENT: [*frustrated*] I feel like my dad is always on my case about everything. I just want him to leave me alone and give me a break.

THERAPIST: It sounds like you are wanting more space. (Criterion 1) Could you help me understand more about what having some space from your dad would look like to you? (Criterion 2)

Example 3

CLIENT: [*sad*] I just feel like no one gets it. No one gets *me*.

THERAPIST: We're all human—no wonder you need to feel understood. (Criterion 1) Can you picture getting this need met? What would someone need to do or say for you to feel really understood? (Criterion 2)

INSTRUCTIONS FOR EXERCISE 5
Step 1: Role-Play and Feedback
• The client says the first beginner client statement. The therapist **improvises** a response based on the skill criteria. • The trainer (or, if not available, the client) provides **brief** feedback based on the skill criteria. • The client then repeats the same statement, and the therapist again improvises a response. The trainer (or client) again provides brief feedback.
Step 2: Repeat
• Repeat Step 1 for all the statements **in the current difficulty** level (beginner, intermediate, or advanced).
Step 3: Assess and Adjust Difficulty
• The therapist completes the Deliberate Practice Reaction Form (see Appendix A) and decides whether to make the exercise easier or harder or to repeat the same difficulty level.
Step 4: Repeat for Approximately 15 Minutes
• Repeat Steps 1 to 3 for at least 15 minutes. • The trainees then switch therapist and client roles and start over.

Now it's your turn! Follow Steps 1 and 2 from the instructions.

Remember: The goal of the role-play is for trainees to practice improvising responses to the client statements in a manner that (a) uses the skill criteria and (b) feels authentic for the trainee. **Example therapist responses for each client statement are provided at the end of this exercise. Trainees should attempt to improvise their own responses before reading the example responses.**

BEGINNER-LEVEL CLIENT STATEMENTS FOR EXERCISE 5
Beginner Client Statement 1
[Frustrated] I'm losing my mind trying to figure out how to be a decent parent, partner, boss, and friend all at the same time. I just want someone to acknowledge how impossible this all is.
Beginner Client Statement 2
[Sad] I feel like my stepmom doesn't care about me. She is always on my case about school and chores.
Beginner Client Statement 3
[Exasperated] I wish I could vent and just let it all out sometimes.
Beginner Client Statement 4
[Lonely] I just feel so disconnected from my girlfriend. I know she's busy, but I don't feel like a priority, and I miss her.
Beginner Client Statement 5
[Uncertain] I don't know what to say when my grandma keeps asking me how I am. My father just got sent up to jail and I don't know what to feel. The way she keeps asking me about it is making it all worse. I know she cares, but I wish she would just leave me alone.

 Assess and adjust the difficulty before moving to the next difficulty level (see Step 3 in the exercise instructions).

INTERMEDIATE-LEVEL CLIENT STATEMENTS FOR EXERCISE 5
Intermediate Client Statement 1
[Overwhelmed] Ever since finding out that my dad isn't my biological dad, I feel like my whole family is a lie. What else aren't they telling me? Why did my mom hide it for so long? Why didn't she think I deserved to know sooner?
Intermediate Client Statement 2
[Sad] My partner keeps acting like nothing happened, but something did happen. I know I was only 8 weeks pregnant, but I can't stop thinking about my miscarriage and what could have been. He just wants to just keep moving forward, but I'm just not there right now.
Intermediate Client Statement 3
[Depressed] No one in our group wants to talk about my friend's death. Why can't we just say it was a suicide?!
Intermediate Client Statement 4
[Annoyed] I don't understand why my mom doesn't get it. I don't want to go to college. I don't want to be a miserable accountant like her.
Intermediate Client Statement 5
[Frustrated] I just want to talk to my brother like we used to without it turning into a political argument.

 Assess and adjust the difficulty before moving to the next difficulty level (see Step 3 in the exercise instructions).

ADVANCED-LEVEL CLIENT STATEMENTS FOR EXERCISE 5
Advanced Client Statement 1
[**Matter-of-factly**] I don't have that much time left. I'm dying, and no one in my family will talk about it. They all just act like the doctors are magicians and somehow this cancer is just going to disappear, but it's not going to happen like that. We can't keep avoiding this.
Advanced Client Statement 2
[**Scared**] It happened again last night. My boyfriend and I were watching TV last night, and there was character whose voice sounded like the guy that raped me. I tried to push it out of my mind and just focus on enjoying the time with him, but I felt myself getting more and more anxious. He tried to ask me if I was OK, and I ended up starting a fight with him about the laundry he left out. I pushed him away like I always do.
Advanced Client Statement 3
[**Nervous**] I'm really scared about coming out to my dad. I know he'll always love me, but I don't know if he'll be able to understand what it means that I'm trans.
Advanced Client Statement 4
[**Depressed**] I wish I mattered to my kids. It feels like now that they are grown, they have no use for me anymore.
Advanced Client Statement 5
[**Dejected**] I'm so lonely.

 Assess and adjust the difficulty here (see Step 3 in the exercise instructions). If appropriate, follow the instructions to make the exercise even more challenging (see Appendix A).

Example Therapist Responses: Helping the Client to Describe Their Distress and Need for Support

Remember: Trainees should attempt to improvise their own responses before reading the example responses. **Do not read the following responses verbatim unless you are having trouble coming up with your own!**

EXAMPLE RESPONSES TO BEGINNER-LEVEL CLIENT STATEMENTS FOR EXERCISE 5
Example Response to Beginner Client Statement 1
With all of the responsibilities you're juggling it makes sense that you need someone to acknowledge and appreciate that. (Criterion 1) What would it look like for someone to meaningfully acknowledge all you are doing? (Criterion 2)
Example Response to Beginner Client Statement 2
It sounds like you really want to feel more care and love from your stepmom. (Criterion 1) What could she do to show you she cares? (Criterion 2)
Example Response to Beginner Client Statement 3
I appreciate you sharing with me here in therapy, but it's completely understandable that you need to share your emotions and experiences with other people—that's what we'll be working on helping you to do. (Criterion 1) Please help me understand what it would look and sound like—in detail—for someone to give you the space to express yourself. (Criterion 2)
Example Response to Beginner Client Statement 4
I'm hearing you say that you need to find ways to connect with your girlfriend that are also respectful of her schedule. (Criterion 1) What have those moments of connection between the two of you looked like in the past? (Criterion 2)
Example Response to Beginner Client Statement 5
It sounds like your grandma really cares but is not yet understanding the room you need to process all that you're going through. (Criterion 1) How could she give you room and still check in with you in ways that wouldn't feel overwhelming to you? What could she say specifically? (Criterion 2)

EXAMPLE RESPONSES TO INTERMEDIATE-LEVEL CLIENT STATEMENTS FOR EXERCISE 5
Example Response to Intermediate Client Statement 1
I hear you saying you still have many questions and need some more clarity—that's understandable given what you are going through. (Criterion 1) Tell me more about what specifically would help give you some more clarity on the situation with your family. (Criterion 2)
Example Response to Intermediate Client Statement 2
It sounds like you need him to understand how big of a loss this is for you, and to be able to walk through it together. (Criterion 1) What exactly do you need him to understand about how you are feeling about the miscarriage to do that? (Criterion 2)
Example Response to Intermediate Client Statement 3
I hear you saying that you want to have honest conversations about what happened. (Criterion 1) Please help me understand more about the things you want to talk to your friends about, and what it would look like for them to support you as you are trying to cope with your friend's suicide. (Criterion 2)
Example Response to Intermediate Client Statement 4
It sounds like you want your mom to understand your own hopes for your future rather than putting you into a box with no options. (Criterion 1) Tell me more about what you would like her to understand about how you are approaching your future. (Criterion 2)
Example Response to Intermediate Client Statement 5
What I hear you saying is that you want to be able to connect meaningfully with your brother. (Criterion 1) What did those moments of connection with him look like in the past? What would need to happen for that connection to be rebuilt? (Criterion 2)

EXAMPLE RESPONSES TO ADVANCED-LEVEL CLIENT STATEMENTS FOR EXERCISE 5

Example Response to Advanced Client Statement 1

It sounds like you need to have the reality of what is happening for you acknowledged rather than people avoiding it. (Criterion 1) Please describe for me more about what it would look like for your family to meaningfully acknowledge what is happening to you, and what you want to be able to talk with them about more specifically. (Criterion 2)

Example Response to Advanced Client Statement 2

I think I hear you saying that you want to find ways to stay connected with him when your trauma response is triggered. (Criterion 1) As you reflect on last night, what would it have looked like for him to support you in that moment in ways that felt safe and supportive to you? (Criterion 2)

Example Response to Advanced Client Statement 3

It's clear that it's important to you to feel your dad's love and acceptance when you share this big part of who you are with him. That's part of being human—we all need love and acceptance. (Criterion 1) In this case, what could your dad do to make you feel safe and show his love and acceptance to you even if he doesn't understand things fully? (Criterion 2)

Example Response to Advanced Client Statement 4

Just so I'm clear, I think I'm hearing you say that you need to feel loved and appreciated by your kids at this point in their lives—at this point in your life too. (Criterion 1) What ideas do you have about what it could look like for them to show you how much they love and care about you now? (Criterion 2)

Example Response to Advanced Client Statement 5

You need to feel meaningfully connected—just like everyone does. (Criterion 1) Can you picture getting this need met? Tell me about what it would look like in practice to feel connected—what do you need from other people to feel that way? (Criterion 2)

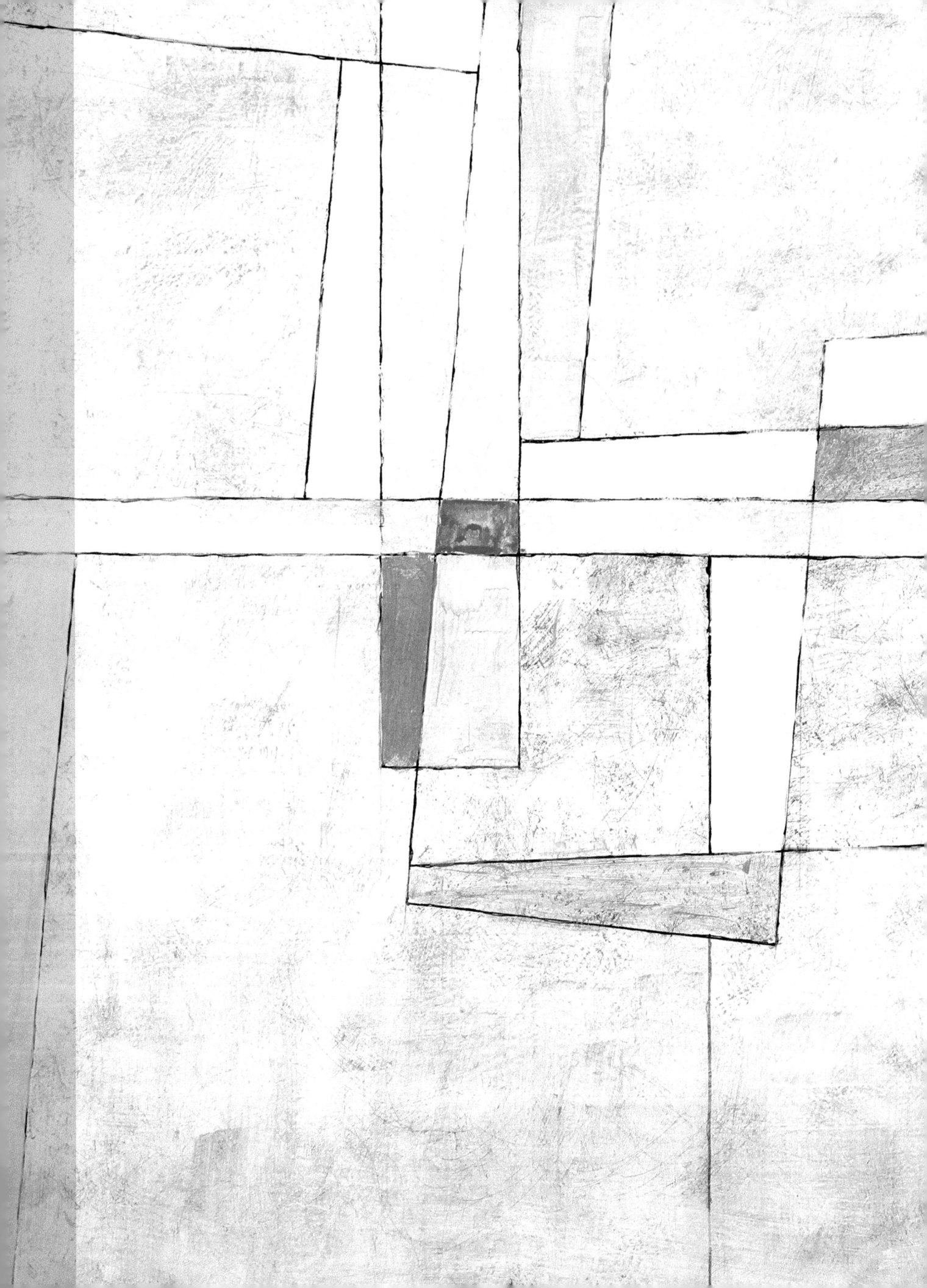

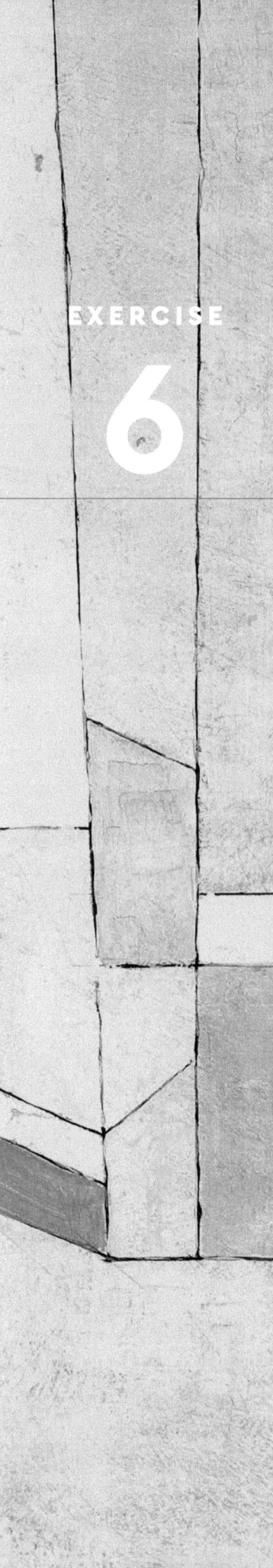

Reinforcement of Effective Communication

Preparations for Exercise 6

1. Read the instructions in Chapter 2.

2. Download the Deliberate Practice Reaction Form and the Deliberate Practice Diary Form at https://www.apa.org/pubs/books/deliberate-practice-interpersonal-psychotherapy (see the "Resources" tab; also available in Appendixes A and B, respectively).

Skill Description

Skill Difficulty Level: Intermediate

Reinforcement of effective communication is a skill that helps identify and expand on the client's good communication in session as a way to encourage more of this communication outside of therapy. Because interpersonal psychotherapy (IPT) is designed to alleviate distress by helping clients strengthen social support and improve interpersonal functioning in their life outside of therapy, good communication is key. The IPT therapist can use their in-session interactions with clients using this skill to provide feedback and motivate effective communication with people in the client's Interpersonal Circle.

As clients are encouraged to share their experiences of distress and needs for support in session, the therapist can model ways to communicate more effectively, particularly using the skills of clarification. The therapist can also provide direct commentary on the patient's communication, using the sessions as a safe laboratory for clients to learn more effective communication strategies and then to practice them. As with any behavioral change—in this case change in communication—the most effective way to effect change is to shape it by reinforcing the positive.

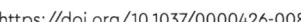

https://doi.org/10.1037/0000426-008

Deliberate Practice in Interpersonal Psychotherapy, by O. Belik, J. M. Schultz, S. Fairhurst, S. Stuart, A. Vaz, and T. Rousmaniere

The skill of interpersonal reinforcement of effective communication helps the clinician provide explicit feedback to clients on their effective communications in session, reinforces the power of the specific communication, and prompts the client to consider how they might use the communication in relationships outside of therapy. The ultimate goal of this skill is to help the patient generalize effective communication skills from the laboratory of therapy to the outside world.

The therapist should improvise a response to each client statement following these skill criteria:

1. **Identify the client's effective use of interpersonal communication in session.** The therapist begins by recognizing and labeling effective client communication in session, including verbal and nonverbal communication. Importantly, it must be effective communication from the client: It should clearly express the client's perspective in a gracious manner that can be heard and understood by others. The therapist should seek to be as explicit as possible in identifying the effective behavioral aspects of the communication. A typical response might be, "That was a beautiful description of the conflict you are having with your partner. The metaphor you used—describing the conflict like an unending siege was really effective in communicating what it has been like for you."

2. **Reinforce how this effective communication positively affects their ability to be understood by the therapist.** It is important for clients to understand how their communication impacts the ability of others in their life to understand their distress and to respond by providing support to them. In this component of the skill, the therapist directly links the client's effective communication in-session to the therapist's own understanding of the client experience. This feedback should be focused on the specifics of the client's effective in-session communication and should reinforce the client's communication behavior, making it more likely that the client will continue to use the demonstrated communication strategy. A typical comment might be, "When you described just now how disappointed you were in your partner, I felt that I really understood even better what that is like for you. The emotion in your voice was really effective in conveying that."

3. **Suggest further use of effective communication strategies outside of session.** The goal of IPT is to strengthen social support and interpersonal functioning in the client's life outside of therapy. Therefore, this skill ends with shifting focus back to relationships in the client's life by graciously suggesting that the client can also use this same communication strategy effectively with others. The therapist may highlight a specific relationship or elicit the client's ideas about whom they envision using the demonstrated communication—for example, "Since I felt like I understood your conflict much better when you described it using that metaphor, I can't help but think that your partner would too. How might you say that to him?"

SKILL CRITERIA FOR EXERCISE 6

1. Identify the client's effective use of interpersonal communication in session.
2. Reinforce how this effective communication positively affects their ability to be understood by the therapist.
3. Suggest further use of effective communication strategies outside of session.

Examples of Therapists Reinforcing Effective Communication

Example 1

CLIENT: [*sad*] I feel like my partner doesn't understand how hard this change is for me. I feel like we've lost our old life together. I'm happy that our family has grown and I love our son, but I also miss the time she and I used to have—just the two of us laughing and talking and doing things together. Sometimes I get angry at her because I miss that.

THERAPIST: I appreciate you sharing how you have been feeling in such an authentic way. (Criterion 1) The way you described it helps me better understand how hard this has been for you. (Criterion 2) I wonder how she would respond if you shared this with her like you just did with me? (Criterion 3)

Example 2

CLIENT: [*sad*] I know I'm supposed to be happy around the holidays, and I do like the lights and the music and the food. But I'm sad. I miss my dad and the way he used to make things magical this time of year. He would always cover my door with wrapping paper on Christmas morning and make a trail of reindeer tracks in the snow in our yard, even when I was in high school. He always made it all so special . . . but he's not here anymore.

THERAPIST: Thanks for sharing that beautiful story with me. (Criterion 1) The way you told it gives me a real sense of how much your dad loved you and cared for you, and it helps me better understand how deep this loss is for you. (Criterion 2) Who else can you share those holiday memories of your dad with? (Criterion 3)

Example 3

CLIENT: [*tearfully and with gratitude*] Thanks for letting me cry. It feels good to let it out a bit. I never do that anywhere else because I have to be strong for my family.

THERAPIST: You're welcome. I'm touched by your bravery in sharing your tears with me. (Criterion 1) I feel like I can understand what this has been like for you when you allow me to experience what you are really feeling in this deep, genuine way. (Criterion 2) I wonder if there are others in your life who could also understand you on this level and would be willing to be with you in the tears. (Criterion 3)

INSTRUCTIONS FOR EXERCISE 6

Step 1: Role-Play and Feedback

- The client says the first beginner client statement. The therapist **improvises** a response based on the skill criteria.
- The trainer (or, if not available, the client) provides **brief** feedback based on the skill criteria.
- The client then repeats the same statement, and the therapist again improvises a response. The trainer (or client) again provides brief feedback.

Step 2: Repeat

- Repeat Step 1 for all the statements **in the current difficulty level** (beginner, intermediate, or advanced).

Step 3: Assess and Adjust Difficulty

- The therapist completes the Deliberate Practice Reaction Form (see Appendix A) and decides whether to make the exercise easier or harder or to repeat the same difficulty level.

Step 4: Repeat for Approximately 15 Minutes

- Repeat Steps 1 to 3 for at least 15 minutes.
- The trainees then switch therapist and client roles and start over.

> **Now it's your turn! Follow Steps 1 and 2 from the instructions.**

Remember: The goal of the role-play is for trainees to practice improvising responses to the client statements in a manner that (a) uses the skill criteria and (b) feels authentic for the trainee. **Example therapist responses for each client statement are provided at the end of this exercise. Trainees should attempt to improvise their own responses before reading the examples.**

BEGINNER-LEVEL CLIENT STATEMENTS FOR EXERCISE 6
Beginner Client Statement 1
[Upset] I called my friend again last week and left another message, but I still haven't heard back. I thought we were close, but no response from her makes me question that. It hurts my feelings. I keep worrying that I did something wrong, worrying if she's okay, or even if something bad happened to her. I get that she's got a lot going on and might not have time for a long phone call. . . . I just need her to send a quick text to let me know she got my message and that she's OK.
Beginner Client Statement 2
[Determined] It's really hard for me to be getting older and to need more help—I don't like to ask for help. I'm grateful for the ways my family is trying to take care of me, but sometimes I wish they would remember I'm still my own person. Even if I do need them for help with rides and housework, I can still make my own decisions about my life. I feel bad even saying this, though, because I worry that I sound ungrateful.
Beginner Client Statement 3
[Overwhelmed] I feel so much pressure to keep it together in front of my wife. I'm the man and I'm supposed to be strong for our family just like my dad was strong for me. Inside, I'm freaking out. My mind is always racing about bills, and rent, and what happens if I get laid off again, and when the car is going to break down, and how we're going to pay for clothes for the kids, and what if one of us needs to go to the doctor. Most days I feel like I'm going to crack under the pressure.
Beginner Client Statement 4
[Frustrated] I asked my mom to teach me to make tortillas, but she keeps telling me that she doesn't have time and that I should just go to the store to buy some. I feel like she doesn't care. My abuela always made tortillas for us, and she always had time for me. She started to teach me how to make them before she died, but I don't remember a lot of it. I really wish I would've paid attention then so I could make them like she used to. I miss abuela so much, and I feel like making tortillas would help me feel close to her again.
Beginner Client Statement 5
[With gratitude] Thanks for asking me questions about my son. I appreciate you listening to my stories and memories. It feels good to talk about him and better days. Everyone else avoids talking about him since his overdose.

 Assess and adjust the difficulty before moving to the next difficulty level (see Step 3 in the exercise instructions).

INTERMEDIATE-LEVEL CLIENT STATEMENTS FOR EXERCISE 6
Intermediate Client Statement 1
[Longingly] I know my parents have been through a lot and sacrificed so much for me to grow up here. They wanted a better life for me than they had, and they risked it all to come to this country. I know they love me, but sometimes I get angry and don't always treat them very nice. It's just that I need them to know that I'm my own person. I want to make them proud, but I want to follow my own path just like they did. I feel so anxious all the time that I'll either let them down or let myself down.
Intermediate Client Statement 2
[Intentionally] Last week was really hard. I need some help today to figure out what to do when the bad thoughts come back again.
Intermediate Client Statement 3
[Overwhelmed] Last night I was washing dishes when my boyfriend got home. I didn't hear him come in the door and all of a sudden I felt someone's arms around me. I freaked out when all he was trying to do was hug me. All these memories from the abuse in my last relationship came flooding back to me, and it was really hard for me to separate what happened then from where I am now. I love my boyfriend, and he makes me feel so safe. It's just in those moments that I feel surprised that I shut down. I know he means well and loves me. This isn't his fault. Why can't I get this under control?
Intermediate Client Statement 4
[Carefully] You said you hear sadness in my voice, but I'm not sure that quite captures how I'm actually feeling. It's more than that . . . I guess I'd describe it more like feeling deflated and hopeless about my brother's addiction.
Intermediate Client Statement 5
[With sadness] I'm so angry at my mom. She went into my room when I was at school and threw away a bunch of stuff, including the Styrofoam cup on my nightstand. It was from the last baseball game I went to with my dad before he got arrested. When we were in line at the concession stand that day, he told me about how he used to go to baseball games with his dad and how much he liked going to baseball games with me. Then he told me how much he loved me. Maybe it's dumb, but seeing that cup in my room made me feel connected to my dad. Now it's gone, and my mom keeps asking me why I'm mad about a "silly cup."

 Assess and adjust the difficulty before moving to the next difficulty level (see Step 3 in the exercise instructions).

ADVANCED-LEVEL CLIENT STATEMENTS FOR EXERCISE 6
Advanced Client Statement 1
[With curiosity] After what we talked about in our appointment last week, I tried being more honest about my expectations with my partner. I think it went alright overall, but I'm not sure how to make sense of something she said. I'd like to talk about it with you today so I can get your feedback.
Advanced Client Statement 2
[Tearfully] I know that I haven't been open with my husband, and I need to. I guess I'm scared about how he'll respond to me. I just need to know he will listen and not judge me.
Advanced Client Statement 3
[Thoughtfully] I'm sorry for laughing when you asked about the fight with my dad. I'm not sure why but sometimes I laugh when I get upset. I'm actually really hurt by the things he said to me.
Advanced Client Statement 4
[Tearfully] Suicide has always been an unspeakable topic in my family, especially because of our religion. I feel like my brother's suicide crushed my heart and put a gag over my mouth. I want to talk about it, but I can't do it.
Advanced Client Statement 5
[Softly, with sadness] I'm lonely, and I worry that my hard exterior pushes people away.

🤚 **Assess and adjust the difficulty here (see Step 3 in the exercise instructions). If appropriate, follow the instructions to make the exercise even more challenging (see Appendix A).**

Example Therapist Responses: Reinforcement of Effective Communication

Remember: Trainees should attempt to improvise their own responses before reading the examples. **Do not read the following responses verbatim unless you are having trouble coming up with your own responses!**

EXAMPLE RESPONSES TO BEGINNER-LEVEL CLIENT STATEMENTS FOR EXERCISE 6
Example Response to Beginner Client Statement 1
I appreciate how honestly you're describing your feelings while also showing empathy for your friend. (Criterion 1) Hearing you talk about it like that helps me understand how difficult it is for you to not hear back from her. (Criterion 2) How could you share this with your friend with that same honesty and empathy? (Criterion 3)
Example Response to Beginner Client Statement 2
I appreciate you so clearly stating your gratitude for their help alongside your need for them to still respect your autonomy. (Criterion 1) Your gracious framing of it like that helps me understand how much this is weighing on you. (Criterion 2) I wonder if we might talk about how you could share both this gratitude and your need for autonomy with your children in ways that they can better understand your experience too. (Criterion 3)
Example Response to Beginner Client Statement 3
What a powerful way to describe how you are really feeling inside. (Criterion 1) Hearing about the pressure you feel to be strong despite the big concerns you have helps me better understand the weight of what you are carrying every day. (Criterion 2) I wonder how your wife would respond if you shared how you are feeling in this way with her. (Criterion 3)
Example Response to Beginner Client Statement 4
Your relationship with your abuela sounds very special—it still is. When you share the reason for wanting to learn to make tortillas as a way to feel connected to her like you just did, (Criterion 1) it helps me understand how important this is to you and why you're wanting to learn from and connect with your mom. (Criterion 2) How could you share the story you just told me with your mom too so that she can better understand why this is so important for you? (Criterion 3)
Example Response to Beginner Client Statement 5
You're welcome. I appreciate you being so clear just now about how helpful it is to you to share those stories and memories with someone. (Criterion 1) That helps me understand why you need that kind of support. (Criterion 2) I wonder how others might respond if you let them know that too? (Criterion 3)

EXAMPLE RESPONSES TO INTERMEDIATE-LEVEL CLIENT STATEMENTS FOR EXERCISE 6

Example Response to Intermediate Client Statement 1

Thanks for sharing your experience in such a beautiful way. (Criterion 1) I can feel and understand your deep emotions when you speak in such a clear way like that. (Criterion 2) I wonder how you could share that level of emotion and insight about what things are like for you with your parents. (Criterion 3)

Example Response to Intermediate Client Statement 2

I'm sorry to hear it was a difficult week for you. I also really appreciate you being so clear and intentional in asking for help with coping today. (Criterion 1) That helps me understand how I can best support you. (Criterion 2) As we talk about coping with the bad thoughts today, I wonder if we might also explore how you can use that kind of direct communication to also ask others in your life for the support you need from them. (Criterion 3)

Example Response to Intermediate Client Statement 3

I'm sorry that happened. You described so clearly your love for your boyfriend alongside how this way of showing affection is so difficult for you. Holding both of those things at the same time is hard. (Criterion 1) The way you shared that helps me understand what happens for you in those moments when you're caught off guard, and your reaction makes sense given what happened. (Criterion 2) What would it feel like to you if you shared this with your boyfriend like you just did with me? (Criterion 3)

Example Response to Intermediate Client Statement 4

Gosh, deflated and hopeless does feel bigger than sadness. I appreciate you gently clarifying that for me—giving me that kind of clear feedback helps me more deeply understand your experience. (Criteria 1 and 2) I wonder how you might be able to share that same kind of feedback with others too so they can better understand what this has really been like for you. (Criterion 3)

Example Response to Intermediate Client Statement 5

It sounds like that was a beautiful day with your dad. When you share the story of the cup with me in that way, it helps me understand what it really means to you and why you're feeling what you're feeling. (Criteria 1 and 2) I'm really sorry it's gone. I wonder how your mom might respond if you told her the story you just shared with me about what that cup meant to you. (Criterion 3)

EXAMPLE RESPONSES TO ADVANCED-LEVEL CLIENT STATEMENTS FOR EXERCISE 6

Example Response to Advanced Client Statement 1

Great job on having that conversation with your partner. I also appreciate you being so clear and direct with me about how you want to use our time together today. (Criterion 1) That really helps me understand what you need from me. (Criterion 2) I want to hear more about the conversation you had with her, and as a part of that, I wonder if we might also explore how you can continue to be open about your needs with your partner like you just did with me. (Criterion 3)

Example Response to Advanced Client Statement 2

Thank you for being so open with me about the fear you are feeling and what you need from your husband. I also appreciate your bravely trusting me with your tears. (Criterion 1) It really helps me understand how you're feeling and what you need when you express it in such a clear and open way. (Criterion 2) What are your ideas about how you could move toward doing that with your husband to let him know how you are feeling about being more vulnerable and what you need from him? (Criterion 3)

Example Response to Advanced Client Statement 3

Thanks for explaining your reaction to me. (Criterion 1) That was really helpful—I was confused about your reaction until you explained it so well. That will be really helpful to understand your reactions moving forward too. (Criterion 2) I wonder if there are times when your reaction might be confusing to others too, and if there might be opportunities to explain to them how you are really feeling, just like you did to me. (Criterion 3)

Example Response to Advanced Client Statement 4

That is such a powerful way to describe what you are going through. (Criterion 1) Those metaphors give me a much deeper sense of the pain you're carrying and how brave you are to try to talk about it more with me. (Criterion 2) I wonder who else might connect with your experience if you framed it in that powerful way? (Criterion 3)

Example Response to Advanced Client Statement 5

What a brave thing to say. The way you shared that with me so honestly and with a soft, open tone of voice helps me connect to how you are really feeling. (Criteria 1 and 2) What would it be like for you to speak with that openness to others? (Criterion 3)

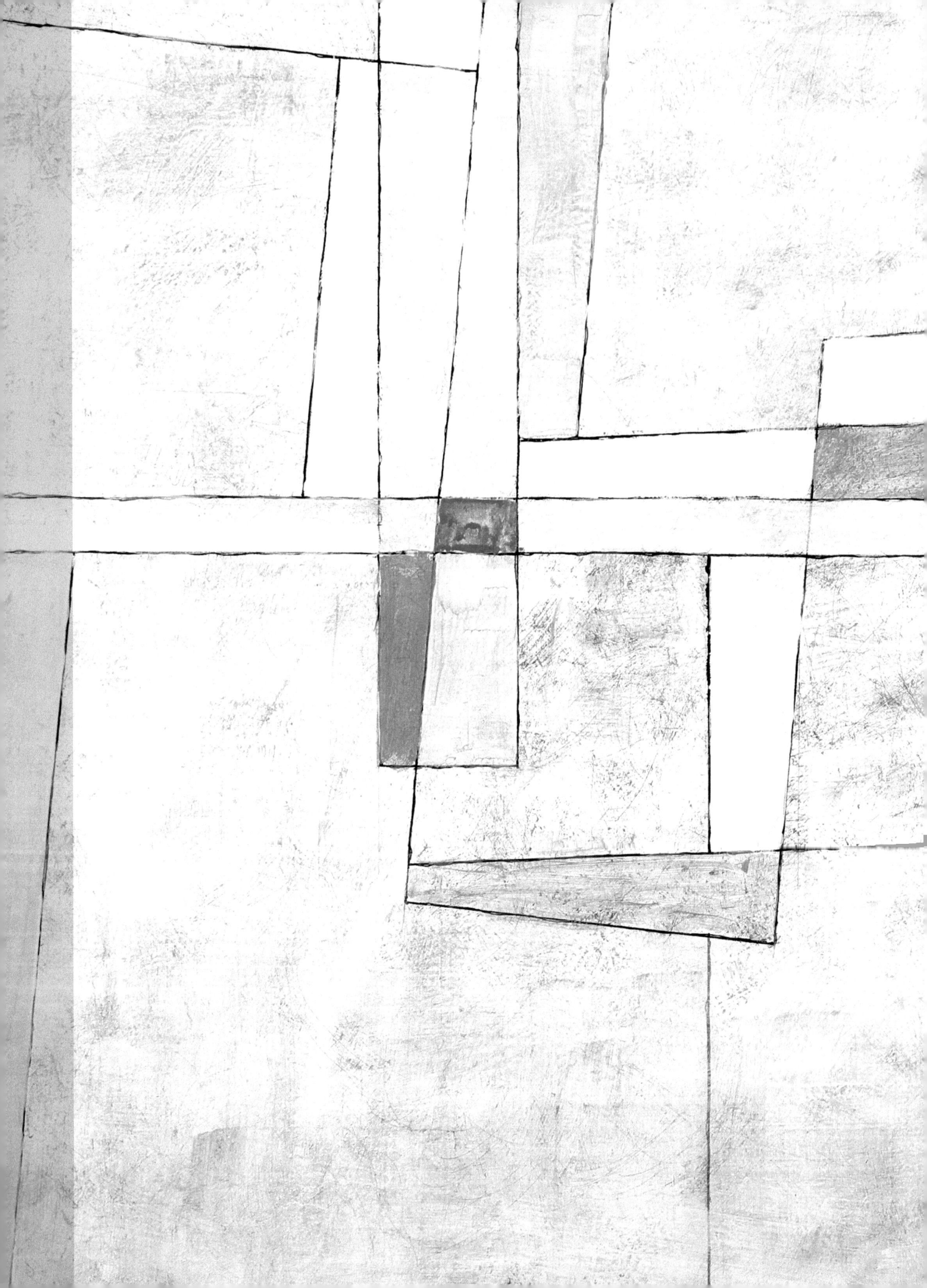

Communication Analysis

Preparations for Exercise 7

1. Read the instructions in Chapter 2.

2. Download the Deliberate Practice Reaction Form and the Deliberate Practice Diary Form at https://www.apa.org/pubs/books/deliberate-practice-interpersonal-psychotherapy (see the "Resources" tab; also available in Appendixes A and B, respectively).

Skill Description

Skill Difficulty Level: Advanced

Our clients often find themselves feeling lonely, frustrated, angry, hopeless, ashamed or confused with the mismatch between their hopes and their experience of their relationships with others they are looking to for support. In interpersonal psychotherapy (IPT), a key activity on a client's path to improvement is engaging their social network, and one of the most useful skills in that journey is to be able to communicate well.

Effective support depends on effective communication. Improved communication leads to greater understanding from others, helping the client feel understood and supported, factors that can lift spirits and even, for those in the deepest of depressions, save a life. The Interpersonal Inventory is the who of social support, occurring in the initial/assessment phase of treatment, while communication analysis is the "how" of social support and occurs in the middle phase.

Communication analysis is accomplished by the therapist assuming a facilitative and curious stance to guide the client through a series of four steps.

https://doi.org/10.1037/0000426-009

Deliberate Practice in Interpersonal Psychotherapy, by O. Belik, J. M. Schultz, S. Fairhurst, S. Stuart, A. Vaz, and T. Rousmaniere

Step 1: Recreate an Interpersonal Incident

An interpersonal incident is a re-creation of a specific interaction, usually one in which the client is asking for support and includes all the verbal and nonverbal communication between the client and their significant other. The incident should include a description of context, place, time, and others who may have been present and should describe the interaction in detail from start to finish. A good analogy is that the interpersonal incident should help the therapist (and client) see and hear the interaction as if it were being rerun on television. The therapist needs good and accurate examples of communication to analyze them.

The specific incidents collected early in therapy usually focus on interactions in which the client asked for support but did not get their needs met. In IPT, the relational frame conceptualization makes clear that problematic communication **always occurs within a system**—it is never the "fault" of one person or another but rather the interactive communication within a system.

The collection of an interpersonal incident may take varying degrees of therapist activity or direction. Although some clients may be naturally good at telling a story or re-creating a dialogue, others may need coaching and direction to recount all of the details. Asking clarifying questions and empathically highlighting the distress the client was experiencing in that interpersonal incident will help the client recognize their emotional experiences throughout the specific interaction. This often involves asking the client directly about the emotions they experienced through each phase of the interaction.

Step 2: Identify Emotions Experienced During the Interpersonal Incident

As we help the client to recall the details of the interpersonal incident, we not only ask the client what happened, who said what, and how each person responded in return, we also help the client gain awareness of their feelings that were emerging during the interpersonal incident. Helping the client understand how communication influenced their feelings during the interpersonal incident will provide the client with additional clarity about the interpersonal occurrence. Specifically, it will highlight how their emotional states influenced their ability to communicate clearly and directly. Identification of emotional states during different phases of the interpersonal incident could lead the client to identify the discrepancy between what they were hoping to feel, what they were hoping to say and gain during the interpersonal incident, and what occurred in reality. Clarity in therapy tends to speed up the therapeutic process of change.

Step 3: Identify the Expectations and Hopes the Client Had During an Interpersonal Incident

Once several samples are collected and examined, the third step in communication analysis is to help the client describe what they were hoping to get from the specific communication in which they were asking for help but did not get it. The therapist should guide the discussion here, although the client has very legitimate needs for support; the fact that their needs were frustrated leads to the likely conclusion that the communication within the relational system was not going well. If so, then the client can do something about it: They can practice more effective communication in session and then implement that communication with another person once again.

Step 4: Identify the Discrepancy Between Client's Expectations and Implemented Communication (or Communication Approach)

Communication analysis reaches the fourth step with a realization that a change in communication is likely the key to interactions that will be more effective, feel more comfortable, and better match the client's hopes and expectations. This is one of the most important insights that clients can come to in IPT—namely, that the way they are communicating within a relationship is not getting what they need and that as a result they can do something to get their needs met by communicating more effectively. The awareness about the discrepancy between their intention in communication and the impact that their communication had on outcomes could increase client's engagement in treatment and motivation to learn and implement different communication skills next time.

This exercise follows a different format and instructions from the other skills in this book. Client statements and therapist responses follow a content thread or dialogue, so that the therapist can practice a conversational back-and-forth that makes up the skill of communication analysis.

The therapist should improvise a response to each client statement following the provided criterion prompts:

1. **Ask the client for relevant details about a specific interpersonal incident.** The therapist starts by prompting the client to recount a specific interpersonal incident, including details from start to finish. The goal is to understand what is not going well with communication within the interpersonal system. In this exercise, the incident should be one in which the client feels that they did not get their needs met sufficiently. A typical prompt is: "Tell me about a time when you asked for help from your partner but felt you did not get the help you needed. Please tell me what happened in detail."

2. **Ask the client about the emotions they experienced during the interpersonal incident.** Communication comes alive with the inclusion of emotion, which impacts the tone in which a request for help is delivered. Encouraging the client to identify their emotions at the time of the interaction allows the therapist and client to better understand the tone that may have been present. For example, the therapist might say, "Now that we have discussed the dialogue in the interaction with your partner in detail, tell me about the emotions you were experiencing during the discussion. What were you feeling?"

3. **Ask the client what they were hoping to get from the other person in the specific incident.** IPT is based on healthy engagement of support networks. Whether a person is grieving, adjusting to a new role, or in conflict, increased intentionality and more effective communication increases the chances their needs will be met. Asking about the client's hopes and expectations during specific interactions and connecting the fact that their needs were not met with the ineffective communication within the system, leads to insight that if communication can be improved, the client's needs are more likely to be met. A therapist might ask, "What were you expecting from the interaction with your partner? What were you hoping they would do?"

4. **Suggest that communication was not effective for the client's purposes.** In communication analysis, motivation to change is enhanced by increasing an understanding of how the communication did or did not match the client's hopes and expectations. Sometimes this step will require only a gentle suggestion, and other times it may require explicitly stating the mismatch. A typical prompt might be: "It seems like something in your communication didn't lead to your friend realizing how much you missed her."

SKILL CRITERIA FOR EXERCISE 7
1. Ask the client for relevant details about a specific interpersonal incident.
2. Ask the client about the emotions they experienced during the interpersonal incident.
3. Ask the client what they were hoping to get from the other person in the specific incident.
4. Suggest that communication was not effective for the client's purposes.

EXAMPLE OF THERAPISTS USING COMMUNICATION ANALYSIS
CLIENT: [*upset*] I had this big fight with Jana yesterday. I keep thinking about how, when she started to cry, for whatever reason I just left and took a walk around the block. Now she's more mad at me than ever.
CRITERION 1: Ask the client for details on their interpersonal incident.
THERAPIST: Let's push rewind just a bit so we can both have a clear picture of what happened up to the point where you took a walk. Can you tell me exactly what happened?
CLIENT: [*frustrated*] We had a disagreement about our friends. I didn't want to go out with them, but she did. From there, we got into an argument and for some reason things escalated, and she started to cry.
CRITERION 2: Ask the client about the emotions they experienced during the interpersonal incident.
THERAPIST: Thinking back to the moment when you could tell she was just about to cry, what emotions were you feeling?
CLIENT: [*confused*] I felt completely confused. I didn't want to make her sad. I mean, I just like to stay home and watch TV and not go out so much. I could tell she was about to cry but I swear to you, I had no idea why.
CRITERION 3: Ask the client what they were hoping to get from the other person in the specific incident.
THERAPIST: When your confusion led you to leave and take a walk around the block, what did you hope would happen by leaving?
CLIENT: [*sorrowful*] I just wanted her to stop crying. All I could think was, "Maybe if I leave then I won't make her upset anymore."
CRITERION 4: Suggest that communication was not effective for the client's purposes.
THERAPIST: Walking out and around the block communicated something to her but it seems like it backfired, huh?

INSTRUCTIONS FOR EXERCISE 7

Step 1: Role-Play With Therapist Improvisation

- The patient initiates the dialogue by reading the first statement in the initial beginner dialogue, then the patient reads aloud the therapist prompt for the first skill criterion.
- The therapist **improvises** a response following the first skill criterion.
- The patient reads the next statement in the same dialogue, followed by the therapist prompt, and the therapist responds using the second criterion. This continues until the dialogue has been completed.

Step 2: Assess and Adjust Difficulty

- The therapist completes the Deliberate Practice Reaction Form (see Appendix A) and decides whether to make the exercise easier or harder or to repeat the same dialogue.

Step 3: Repeat for Approximately 15 Minutes

- Repeat Steps 1 and 2 for at least 15 minutes.
- The trainees then switch therapist and patient roles and start over.

Now it's your turn! Follow Step 1 from the exercise instructions.

Remember: The goal of the role-play is for trainees to practice improvising responses to the patient statements in a manner that (a) uses the skill criteria and (b) feels authentic for the trainee. **Example clinician responses for each patient statement are provided at the end of this exercise. Trainees should attempt to improvise their own responses before reading the examples.**

BEGINNER-LEVEL DIALOGUE 1
CLIENT: [Sad] My mom and I really haven't talked since she told me about her decision to not get chemo. I mean, me and my kids will be okay, but I don't think she knows how much we'll miss her and now we're not even talking.
THERAPIST PROMPT (CRITERION 1): *Ask the client for details on their interpersonal incident.*
CLIENT: [Gloomy] I said something like, "That's definitely your right," and then she said, "Thank you for respecting that." Then we each said goodbye and hung up.
THERAPIST PROMPT (CRITERION 2): *Ask the client about the emotions they experienced during the interpersonal incident.*
CLIENT: [Sorrowful] I was just sad—sad that she's going to die and maybe even sadder that I don't think she realizes how much we'll miss her.
THERAPIST PROMPT (CRITERION 3): *Ask the client what they were hoping to get from the other person in the specific incident.*
CLIENT: [Frustrated] I was hoping we would talk about how we would spend the time we have left, but now, though, we haven't even talked at all in over a week.
THERAPIST PROMPT (CRITERION 4): *Suggest that communication was not effective for the client's purposes.*

BEGINNER-LEVEL DIALOGUE 2
CLIENT: [Upset] I'm so frustrated that he makes jokes and blows me off when we have to make serious decisions about money.
THERAPIST PROMPT (CRITERION 1): *Ask the client for details on their interpersonal incident.*
CLIENT: [Frustrated] His car needs to go into the shop—again!—and so it looks like we'll have to get a new car, which we probably can't afford. I told him we'd have to cut back on everything but rent and food, and so he said he feels like he lives with a goblin from Gringotts Bank. I told him that he's just hilarious while I looked down at the floor.
THERAPIST PROMPT (CRITERION 2): *Ask the client about the emotions they experienced during the interpersonal incident.*
CLIENT: [Frustrated] I was feeling so frustrated, like he doesn't realize how much effort and planning it takes to make sure our budget works, and so he makes a joke like saying I'm the problem.
THERAPIST PROMPT (CRITERION 3): *Ask the client what they were hoping to get from the other person in the specific incident.*
CLIENT: [Disappointed] I guess I figured he would realize that he'd upset me and that it was a serious issue. I hoped he would say sorry and then ask where we should cut back our spending.
THERAPIST PROMPT (CRITERION 4): *Suggest that communication was not effective for the client's purposes.*

 Assess and adjust the difficulty before moving to the next difficulty level (see Step 2 in the exercise instructions).

INTERMEDIATE-LEVEL DIALOGUE 1

CLIENT: [Disheartened] The last time my friends from high school came to visit I think I depressed them and now they haven't been back for 3 or 4 months.

THERAPIST PROMPT (CRITERION 1): *Ask the client for details on their interpersonal incident.*

CLIENT: [Sad] That's easy because, since the car accident, all I do is lie around the house or go to doctors' appointments. I promised myself I'd talk about something other than back pain and loneliness, but it was all that seemed to come out of my mouth. Then I'd apologize for saying it . . . again and again. I don't even blame them for not coming back.

THERAPIST PROMPT (CRITERION 2): *Ask the client about the emotions they experienced during the interpersonal incident.*

CLIENT: [Discouraged] I've been so lonely since the accident, so discouraged by the pain, but then every time I said it, I was also ashamed.

THERAPIST PROMPT (CRITERION 3): *Ask the client what they were hoping to get from the other person in the specific incident.*

CLIENT: [Disappointed] Honestly, I know I can't do much, so I just wanted to hear them tell fun stories so we could laugh together and I could mentally sort of "escape." Instead, they had to listen to me moan, and now they probably feel too awkward to want to come back.

THERAPIST PROMPT (CRITERION 4): *Suggest that communication was not effective for the client's purposes.*

INTERMEDIATE-LEVEL DIALOGUE 2
CLIENT: [Embarrassed] In front of everyone, including my boss's boss, my first project since the promotion got criticized again and again, and now I'll bet they wonder if they should have any faith in me at all.
THERAPIST PROMPT (CRITERION 1): *Ask the client for details on their interpersonal incident.*
CLIENT: [Uncomfortable] I think I set the record for the number of times people said, "This is why it's so important to involve other departments from the beginning." There must have been 20 people in the meeting, all these higher-ups, and they kept hearing that I had blown it. All I could say, repeatedly, was "Thank you for your feedback."
THERAPIST PROMPT (CRITERION 2): *Ask the client about the emotions they experienced during the interpersonal incident.*
CLIENT: [Hopeless] It was weird. Maybe hopeless or something? I remember sort of feeling dizzy and sick, like I just wanted to leave.
THERAPIST PROMPT (CRITERION 3): *Ask the client what they were hoping to get from the other person in the specific incident.*
CLIENT: [Sad] I was hoping that they would have seen all the work that had been put into the project and that they would be more encouraging.
THERAPIST PROMPT (CRITERION 4): *Suggest that communication was not effective for the client's purposes.*

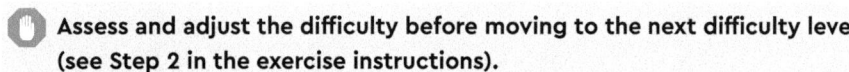 **Assess and adjust the difficulty before moving to the next difficulty level (see Step 2 in the exercise instructions).**

ADVANCED-LEVEL DIALOGUE 1
CLIENT: [Offended] I made one joke and now it's a federal case about whether I'm a fit parent. Everyone knows we shouldn't get a dog when we have a disabled son, I'm just the one who said what everyone should have been thinking.
THERAPIST PROMPT (CRITERION 1): *Ask the client for details on their interpersonal incident.*
CLIENT: [Overwhelmed] My 13-year-old with autism has been nonstop excited about asking for a dog. Since we live with my wife's parents, the house is crowded and our life only works when the routine is strictly followed, so I made the joke that "we'll be the first house ever where the puppy is the one who gets bit by the kid." My son started crying and my father-in-law said maybe I should take some time away from the family.
THERAPIST PROMPT (CRITERION 2): *Ask the client about the emotions they experienced during the interpersonal incident.*
CLIENT: [Confused] I kept thinking, "You've got to be kidding me." Like, how was I the only one who understood that this was a bad idea? That's a feeling, right?
THERAPIST PROMPT (CRITERION 3): *Ask the client what they were hoping to get from the other person in the specific incident.*
CLIENT: [Frustrated] I was hoping that they would see the absurdity of what they were even considering and then realize that we obviously shouldn't get a dog.
THERAPIST PROMPT (CRITERION 4): *Suggest that communication was not effective for the client's purposes.*

ADVANCED-LEVEL DIALOGUE 2
CLIENT: [Annoyed] I need to request a roommate switch. He is talking nonstop about politics, and I've never heard someone so unbearably self-righteous and at the same time so naive and blind about what's really going on.
THERAPIST PROMPT (CRITERION 1): *Ask the client for details on their interpersonal incident.*
CLIENT: [Irritated] Sure. Just yesterday he came back from class and started yelling about everything from taxes to climate change to the upcoming election like anyone who disagreed with him was an idiot. I was reading and just shook my head and said, "Meanwhile, the rest of us have to study." And he said, "Typical," before turning up the volume on his podcast without using the headphones.
THERAPIST PROMPT (CRITERION 2): *Ask the client about the emotions they experienced during the interpersonal incident.*
CLIENT: [Upset] I was feeling angry that I have to put up with this moron.
THERAPIST PROMPT (CRITERION 3): *Ask the client what they were hoping to get from the other person in the specific incident.*
CLIENT: [Confused] That was way more than a hint, right? I was hoping he'd be quiet or that he would go to another room so that I could study in peace.
THERAPIST PROMPT (CRITERION 4): *Suggest that communication was not effective for the client's purposes.*

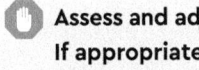 **Assess and adjust the difficulty here (see Step 2 in the exercise instructions). If appropriate, follow the instructions to make the exercise even more challenging (see Appendix A).**

Example Therapist Responses: Communication Analysis

Remember: Trainees should attempt to improvise their own responses before reading the examples. **Do not read the following responses verbatim unless you are having trouble coming up with your own!**

EXAMPLE RESPONSES TO BEGINNER-LEVEL DIALOGUE 1
CLIENT: **[Sad]** My mom and I really haven't talked since she told me about her decision to not get chemo. I mean, me and my kids will be okay, but I don't think she knows how much we'll miss her and now we're not even talking.
THERAPIST: Can you take me back to that conversation and what happened right after she told you her decision?
CLIENT: **[Gloomy]** I said something like, "That's definitely your right," and then she said, "Thank you for respecting that." Then we each said goodbye and hung up.
THERAPIST: After hearing her decision, and maybe just before you said, "It's your right," what were you feeling?
CLIENT: **[Sorrowful]** I was just sad—sad that she's going to die and maybe even sadder that I don't think she realizes how much we'll miss her.
THERAPIST: How were you hoping the conversation would go, especially when you said, "That's definitely your right?"
CLIENT: **[Frustrated]** I was hoping we would talk about how we would spend the time we have left, but now, though, we haven't even talked at all in over a week.
THERAPIST: It seems like something in the communication didn't lead to her realizing how much you and your kids will miss her.

EXAMPLE RESPONSES TO BEGINNER-LEVEL DIALOGUE 2
CLIENT: [Upset] I'm so frustrated that he makes jokes and blows me off when we have to make serious decisions about money.
THERAPIST: Can you think of a time that happened and then tell me, step by step, how it went?
CLIENT: [Frustrated] His car needs to go into the shop—again!—and so it looks like we'll have to get a new car which we probably can't afford. I told him we'd have to cut back on everything but rent and food, and so he said he feels like he lives with a goblin from Gringotts Bank. I told him that he's just hilarious while I looked down at the floor.
THERAPIST: After he made the goblin joke and just before you said he's hilarious, what were you feeling?
CLIENT: [Frustrated] I was feeling so frustrated, like he doesn't realize how much effort and planning it takes to make sure our budget works and so he makes a joke like saying I'm the problem.
THERAPIST: How were you hoping the budget conversation would go, especially after you said, "You're hilarious," and looked at the floor?
CLIENT: [Disappointed] I guess I figured he would realize that he'd upset me and that it was a serious issue. I hoped he would say sorry and then ask where we should cut back our spending?
THERAPIST: It didn't go there though. It sounds like his takeaway was something different.

EXAMPLE RESPONSES TO INTERMEDIATE-LEVEL DIALOGUE 1
CLIENT: **[Disheartened]** The last time my friends from high school came to visit I think I depressed them, and now they haven't been back for 3 or 4 months.
THERAPIST: Can you put your mind back to that day and tell me, step by step, how it went?
CLIENT: **[Sad]** That's easy because, since the car accident, all I do is lie around the house or go to doctors' appointments. I promised myself I'd talk about something other than back pain and loneliness, but it was all that seemed to come out of my mouth. Then I'd apologize for saying it . . . again and again. I don't even blame them for not coming back.
THERAPIST: How were you feeling, specifically when you noticed you were saying the things you had promised yourself you wouldn't say?
CLIENT: **[Discouraged]** I've been so lonely since the accident, so discouraged by the pain, but then every time I said it, I was also ashamed.
THERAPIST: What were you hoping would happen during the visit?
CLIENT: **[Disappointed]** Honestly, I know I can't do much, so I just wanted to hear them tell fun stories so we could laugh together, and I could mentally sort of "escape." Instead, they had to listen to me moan, and now they probably feel too awkward to want to come back.
THERAPIST: It seems that you do need a space to share your emotions and current experiences with someone, but doing it with this group of friends didn't lead to them telling fun stories like you had hoped.

EXAMPLE RESPONSES TO INTERMEDIATE-LEVEL DIALOGUE 2
CLIENT: [Embarrassed] In front of everyone, including my boss's boss, my first project since the promotion got criticized again and again, and now I'll bet they wonder if they should have any faith in me at all.
THERAPIST: I'm sure it will be uncomfortable, but can you push rewind on that meeting and tell me, in some detail, how it went?
CLIENT: [Uncomfortable] I think I set the record for the number of times people said, "This is why it's so important to involve other departments from the beginning." There must have been 20 people in the meeting, all of these higher-ups, and they kept hearing that I had blown it. All I could say, repeatedly, was "Thank you for your feedback."
THERAPIST: Can you describe how you felt, right in that moment before you said, "Thank you for your feedback"?
CLIENT: [Hopeless] It was weird. Maybe hopeless or something? I remember sort of feeling dizzy and sick, like I just wanted to leave.
THERAPIST: How were you hoping that the other people in the meeting would respond when you said, "Thank you for your feedback"?
CLIENT: [Sad] I was hoping that they would have seen all the work that had gone into the project and that they would be more encouraging.
THERAPIST: It sounds like the statement "Thank you for your feedback" didn't end up prompting the meeting in the direction that you had hoped.

EXAMPLE RESPONSES TO ADVANCED-LEVEL DIALOGUE 1
CLIENT: [Offended] I made one joke, and now it's a federal case about whether I'm a fit parent. Everyone knows we shouldn't get a dog when we have a disabled son, I'm just the one who said what everyone should have been thinking.
THERAPIST: Can you tell me, in more detail, about the conversation, the joke you made, and how people reacted?
CLIENT: [Overwhelmed] My 13-year-old with autism has been nonstop excited about asking for a dog. Since we live with my wife's parents, the house is crowded, and our life really only works when the routine is strictly followed, so I made the joke that "we'll be the first house ever where the puppy is the one who gets bit by the kid." My son started crying and my father-in-law said maybe I should take some time away from the family.
THERAPIST: As you were experiencing the family conversation, and right before you made the joke, how were you feeling?
CLIENT: [Confused] I kept thinking, "You've got to be kidding me." Like, how was I the only one who understood that this was a bad idea? That's a feeling, right?
THERAPIST: How were you expecting the others to respond when you made the joke?
CLIENT: [Frustrated] I was hoping that they would see the absurdity of what they were even considering and then realize that we obviously shouldn't get a dog.
THERAPIST: It sounds like different people, from your son to your father-in-law, had a different response than what you were hoping for.

EXAMPLE RESPONSES TO ADVANCED-LEVEL DIALOGUE 2
CLIENT: **[Annoyed]** I need to request a roommate switch. He is talking nonstop about politics, and I've never heard someone so unbearably self-righteous and at the same time so naive and blind about what's really going on.
THERAPIST: Can you tell me, step by step, about a specific interaction where you realized that you might need to switch roommates?
CLIENT: **[Irritated]** Sure. Just yesterday he came back from class and started yelling about everything from taxes to climate change to the upcoming election like anyone who disagreed with him was an idiot. I was reading and just shook my head and said, "Meanwhile, the rest of us have to study." And he said, "Typical," before turning up the volume on his podcast without using the headphones.
THERAPIST: What were you feeling, just before you said, "Meanwhile . . ."?
CLIENT: **[Upset]** I was feeling angry that I have to put up with this moron.
THERAPIST: What were you hoping would happen after you said that you had to study?
CLIENT: **[Confused]** That was way more than a hint, right? I was hoping he'd be quiet or that he would go to another room so that I could study in peace.
THERAPIST: When you said, "Meanwhile, the rest of us have to study," it sounds like he reacted differently than you wanted.

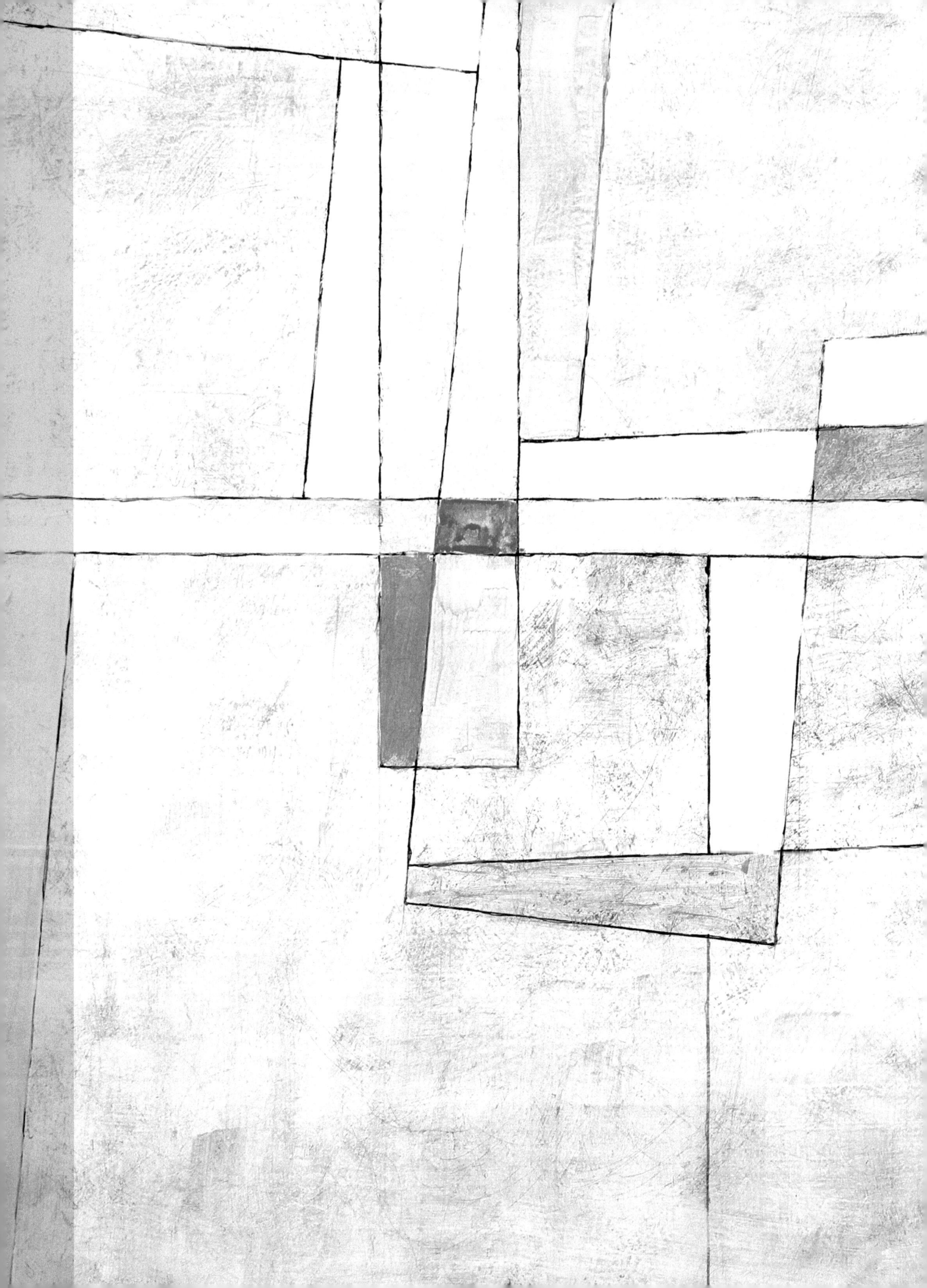

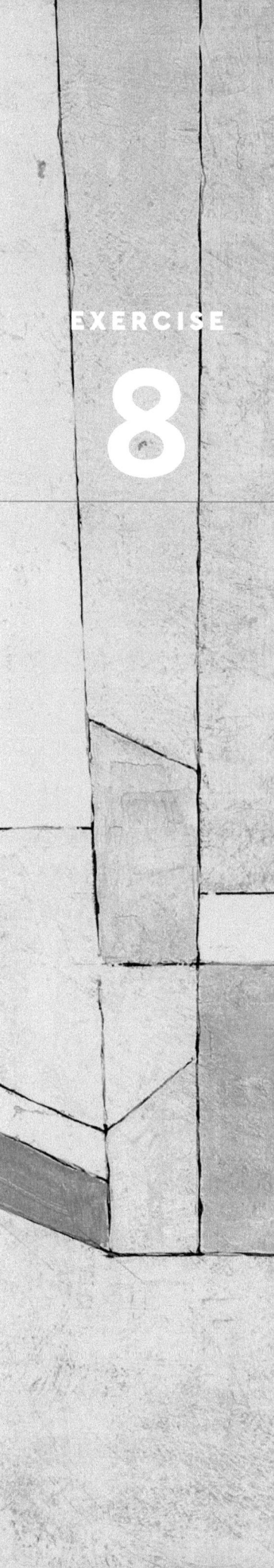

Generating Communication Options

Preparations for Exercise 8

1. Read the instructions in Chapter 2.

2. Download the Deliberate Practice Reaction Form and the Deliberate Practice Diary Form at https://www.apa.org/pubs/books/deliberate-practice-interpersonal-psychotherapy (see the "Resources" tab; also available in Appendixes A and B, respectively).

Skill Description

Skill Difficulty Level: Advanced

The four steps of communication analysis discussed in Exercise 7 help clients become readier to make changes in their life. Collecting interpersonal incidents, helping the client recognize their emotional experiences, and asking them what they are hoping to get from other people in the system are all designed to motivate them to revise how they communicate. That motivation is strengthened by the suggestion from the therapist that improved communication may lead to different results. Communication is a learned skill—clients can be taught to do it well. This chapter covers the next step in the process: helping the client develop communication options and practice them.

As during the rest of interpersonal psychotherapy (IPT), a collaborative approach will be most effective, with the client and therapist both contributing ideas and brainstorming together. On a metalevel, the clinician can use this collaborative approach to model good communication in the session. This modeling can be an effective way to teach the client more effective communication skills.

This skill focuses on facilitating the client's ability to identify and practice suggested options. Modifying suggestions developed by the client, if possible, is nearly always the

https://doi.org/10.1037/0000426-010

Deliberate Practice in Interpersonal Psychotherapy, by O. Belik, J. M. Schultz, S. Fairhurst, S. Stuart, A. Vaz, and T. Rousmaniere

best way to come up with and try out ideas. Doing this also builds the client's confidence and empowers them, as well as teaching more general skills that can be used to deal with future communication problems. The old adage "give a person a fish, and they eat for a day; teach a person to fish, and they will eat for a lifetime" is a good way to describe this. The clinician should reinforce the client's good ideas and refine them through feedback and modeling.

The therapist should improvise a response to each client statement following these skill criteria:

1. **Provide feedback to the client about proposed communication options.** When a client identifies a reasonable option to communicate more effectively, the clinician should reinforce and, when needed, help to refine their proposed idea. One way to do this well is to provide elements of STAR feedback: Supportive, Timely, Actionable, and Relevant. This feedback will also model for the client how to communicate in relationships outside of therapy. *Supportive* feedback identifies an element of the solution, such as "What you just said really shows your compassion." *Timeliness* refers practically to providing feedback right after the client suggests a statement. *Actionable* feedback includes direct suggestions for revisions that might improve the communication further, and *relevant* feedback allows the clinician to reflect on how the communication might be received and acted upon by the intended recipient. This process with a client in therapy mirrors the idea of deliberate practice in this book, and deliberate practice generally.

2. **Practice the proposed communication options using role-playing.** Nearly everyone agrees that "practice makes perfect" (or at least practice improves skills significantly). Nonetheless, many clients are reluctant to engage in the role-playing to do that practicing (a meta-moment not lost on either the writers or readers of this book). In IPT, the clinician can be subtle in moving toward practice and can initiate role-playing by simply beginning to do it. Practically, this means asking the client to reflect on how they would respond to a revised version of the communication that they have already proposed. This kind of "nudge" is a way to influence the communication in therapy, and of course also models ways the client can communicate effectively in relationships outside of therapy as well. A typical prompt to move into role-playing is "The way you just described your irritation with your partner sounded very good to me. How do you think she would respond if you changed it just slightly by starting pleasantly like this: 'I appreciate your help. It would be even more helpful if you could check in with me before you get started on a project so we can think it through together.'"

SKILL CRITERIA FOR EXERCISE 8

1. Provide feedback to the client about their proposed communication options.
2. Practice the proposed communication options using role-playing.

Examples of Therapists Generating Communication Options

Example 1

CLIENT: [*dejected*] Maybe I could just tell Claire that it's hard for me to hear about her job. It's been 6 months since graduation and I'm still unemployed.

THERAPIST: That's a nice and direct way to let her know that you value the friendship and that it's a sensitive topic. (Criterion 1) Okay, imagine you're Claire, and let's see how this lands: "I'm really happy for you, but while I'm still unemployed it's hard for me to talk about your job. Can we talk about other things?" How does that strike you? (Criterion 2)

Example 2

CLIENT: [*disappointed*] I want to tell my son I'm trying to do better, that I'll get him out of foster care and that I'll be sober, but I don't know how to say it to him.

THERAPIST: Your love for him really comes through in what you just said to me. . . . Maybe you can emphasize that love and keep his expectations realistic at the same time. (Criterion 1) How do you think he would respond to this? "I love you. That love is forever. It's been really hard for me to stay sober, but when I finally do, both of our lives will improve a little bit every day." (Criterion 2)

Example 3

CLIENT: [*sad*] I don't want to be a burden, but maybe I could talk to my godmother and let her know, now that my mom's died, that she's going to have to step up with the promises she probably forgot that she made when I was a baby.

THERAPIST: I love how you can be funny, even at the darkest times, and still say what you mean. I'll even guess that your godmother would consider it more an honor than a burden to help care for you. (Criterion 1) Let me try something out. Listen like you're her and just respond like you think she might. "I need you to step up with the promises you probably forgot from when I was a baby. I hope it's okay that I lean on you more if things get hard for me now that my mom's gone." (Criterion 2)

INSTRUCTIONS FOR EXERCISE 8

Step 1: Role-Play and Feedback

- The client says the first beginner client statement. The therapist **improvises** a response based on the skill criteria.
- The trainer (or, if not available, the client) provides **brief** feedback based on the skill criteria.
- The client then repeats the same statement, and the therapist again improvises a response. The trainer (or client) again provides brief feedback.

Step 2: Repeat

- Repeat Step 1 for all the statements **in the current difficulty level** (beginner, intermediate, or advanced).

Step 3: Assess and Adjust Difficulty

- The therapist completes the Deliberate Practice Reaction Form (see Appendix A) and decides whether to make the exercise easier or harder or to repeat the same difficulty level.

Step 4: Repeat for Approximately 15 Minutes

- Repeat Steps 1 to 3 for at least 15 minutes.
- The trainees then switch therapist and client roles and start over.

Now it's your turn! Follow Steps 1 and 2 from the instructions.

Remember: The goal of the role-play is for trainees to practice improvising responses to the client statements in a manner that (a) uses the skill criteria and (b) feels authentic for the trainee. **Example therapist responses for each client statement are provided at the end of this exercise. Trainees should attempt to improvise their own responses before reading the examples.**

BEGINNER-LEVEL CLIENT STATEMENTS FOR EXERCISE 8
Beginner Client Statement 1
[Dejected] Maybe I could tell my friends that I want to hang out again, now that I got dumped.
Beginner Client Statement 2
[Angrily] I want to tell my teenager that he should do more to get better grades, and that starts with spending less time playing video games.
Beginner Client Statement 3
[Irritated] I want to tell her that she shouldn't act superior to her cousins because it's just mean.
Beginner Client Statement 4
[Optimistic] I could try sitting next to someone new in the dining hall instead of taking food to my dorm room.
Beginner Client Statement 5
[Timidly] Even though it would be awkward as the youngest one there, I could join that support group for Parkinson's, "Silver Sneakers," and try not to say something that alienates the group.

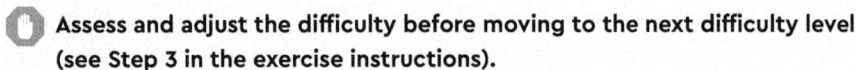 **Assess and adjust the difficulty before moving to the next difficulty level (see Step 3 in the exercise instructions).**

INTERMEDIATE-LEVEL CLIENT STATEMENTS FOR EXERCISE 8
Intermediate Client Statement 1
[Dejected] I should just tell my boss that it's depressing to never get any praise.
Intermediate Client Statement 2
[Lonely] My parents don't need me to be whiny about depression, not with my brother back in the hospital. However, I still need their support.
Intermediate Client Statement 3
[Exhausted] God forgive me, but I probably ought to tell their social worker that I'm just exhausted trying to be a Resource Parent to those twins.
Intermediate Client Statement 4
[Determined] I think my dad will respect me if I tell him, like a man, that I'm gay. I can't believe I'm saying this.
Intermediate Client Statement 5
[Skeptically] I'll probably lose a few friends, but I should tell them that I'm still on probation, wearing an ankle monitor.

🛑 **Assess and adjust the difficulty before moving to the next difficulty level (see Step 3 in the exercise instructions).**

ADVANCED-LEVEL CLIENT STATEMENTS FOR EXERCISE 8
Advanced Client Statement 1
[Self-critically] I'm so ashamed that I cheated. I want to ask my wife for forgiveness but don't know how.
Advanced Client Statement 2
[Irritated] This is probably the wrong thing to say, but I really want to tell him that dealing with being stuck in a wheelchair isn't as hard for me as feeling like I'm a burden on him.
Advanced Client Statement 3
[Depressed] I guess I just want to let my parents know that I love them and that my suicide attempt wasn't their fault.
Advanced Client Statement 4
[Angrily] My neighbor needs to hear it loud and clear that his dog needs to shut up or else.
Advanced Client Statement 5
[Sad] I hope my boyfriend won't love me any less, but I don't think I should keep it a secret any longer. . . . My first child, who's 10 now, was adopted away because of my drug use.

🛑 **Assess and adjust the difficulty here (see Step 3 in the exercise instructions). If appropriate, follow the instructions to make the exercise even more challenging (see Appendix A).**

Example Therapist Responses: Generating Communication Options

Remember: Trainees should attempt to improvise their own responses before reading the examples. **Do not read the following responses verbatim unless you are having trouble coming up with your own!**

EXAMPLE RESPONSES TO BEGINNER-LEVEL CLIENT STATEMENTS FOR EXERCISE 8
Example Response to Beginner Client Statement 1
I'm impressed that you want to engage your friends, and it sounds smart to let them know where you're coming from. (Criterion 1) How would they respond if you said something like **"I know I haven't been around much, but I appreciate our friendship even more after the breakup and would love to hang out."** (Criterion 2)
Example Response to Beginner Client Statement 2
It's hard to sometimes feel like you want more for your teenager than they want for themselves. What you just said is certainly direct, but I wonder how it will be received. (Criterion 1) I wonder how a slight change might work. You listen as if you are your son, and then give me a response: **"I'm concerned about your grades—I want you to do well and I know you have the capability to do well. Let's talk about how we can work together to set a limit on the video-game time so you can accomplish what you want to in school."** (Criterion 2)
Example Response to Beginner Client Statement 3
I'm impressed by you looking out for other people's feelings. I like the direct approach you're considering with your daughter, especially including your values, but I'm thinking that calling her mean might backfire. (Criterion 1) If you were her, how do you think she might respond to this: **"I want to help you to be kind to your cousins because kindness is a value in our family."** (Criterion 2)
Example Response to Beginner Client Statement 4
I know it may not sound like bravery, but that really is a brave suggestion. (Criterion 1) If you were the other person, how might you respond to someone saying, **"Is it okay if I sit here?"** (Criterion 2)
Example Response to Beginner Client Statement 5
No one expects to have to deal with a disease like Parkinson's, and your positive attitude about it is impressive. (Criterion 1) If you were one of the older people and in walks this 50-year-old saying, **"Hi, I'm trying to keep my Parkinson's from catching up with me. Is there room here for one more?,"** what do you think they'd say? (Criterion 2)

EXAMPLE RESPONSES TO INTERMEDIATE-LEVEL
CLIENT STATEMENTS FOR EXERCISE 8

Example Response to Intermediate Client Statement 1

You're smart to communicate directly to your boss about how positive feedback is important in motivating you. Getting positive feedback is important for everyone. (Criterion 1) How about if we consider more of an emphasis on the positives? If you were your boss, how would you respond to this: **"I'm really the kind of person who responds well to good feedback. Let me know what I'm doing well, and I'll do it even more."** (Criterion 2)

Example Response to Intermediate Client Statement 2

You're a really caring person, even looking out for your parents. I think you can get support without being whiny. (Criterion 1) How would they respond if you said, **"I know with Andre back in the hospital that you're both exhausted, but I hope it's still okay for me to come to you for support when I'm feeling down."** (Criterion 2)

Example Response to Intermediate Client Statement 3

I hear what you are saying—you're clear in communicating that you're exhausted. A caring Resource Parent knows when to ask for help. (Criterion 1) If you were the social worker, how would you respond to this: **"I'm feeling more tired than I ever have been, trying to care for the twins. I think I need more help."** (Criterion 2)

Example Response to Intermediate Client Statement 4

You know your dad, and you know yourself. I think you're smart to trust that. (Criterion 1) Give me a sense of how he might respond if you said it just like that: **"Dad, I want to tell you, man to man, that I'm gay."** (Criterion 2)

Example Response to Intermediate Client Statement 5

It's never easy to come clean about something you wish you had done differently in the past, but they may well respect you even more for coming clean just like you suggested. (Criterion 1) What do you think your friends would say if you just communicated it straight up: **"It's hard for me to say this, but I want to be honest and up-front with you. I've got to leave early because I'm still on probation, and because of that, I have a curfew that's monitored. I think it's better that you know than me making up an excuse."** (Criterion 2)

EXAMPLE RESPONSES TO ADVANCED-LEVEL CLIENT STATEMENTS FOR EXERCISE 8

Example Response to Advanced Client Statement 1

Forgiveness is a difficult ask. Your acknowledgment of that difficulty would be a good place to start. (Criterion 1) Putting yourself in her place, how would she respond to this: **"I'm so sorry for what I've done, and I want to ask for your forgiveness. I know this is difficult for both of us, especially for you."** (Criterion 2)

Example Response to Advanced Client Statement 2

Telling him that it's hard for you to feel like you're a burden isn't a "wrong" thing to say, but saying something like that takes some graciousness to go over well. (Criterion 1) Imagining that you're in his place, go ahead and respond to this: **"I really appreciate all of the care you give me, but being in this wheelchair is in some ways easier than me feeling like I'm a burden on you."** (Criterion 2)

Example Response to Advanced Client Statement 3

I know your parents want you to be okay and I appreciate how much you want to make sure that they're also okay—you made that very clear in what you just said. (Criterion 1) Give me a sense of how they might respond if you said it straight: **"I really want you to know that my suicide attempt wasn't your fault and that I love you both."** (Criterion 2)

Example Response to Advanced Client Statement 4

Asserting your right to quiet in the neighborhood is fair but the "or else" might be more trouble than it's worth. (Criterion 1) Let me hear how your neighbor might respond if you said something like, **"I'd really like to have it quiet after 10:00 so I can sleep with the windows open. I'd appreciate it if you would keep your dog quiet or in your house after 10:00."** (Criterion 2)

Example Response to Advanced Client Statement 5

It sounds like for you, and I'll bet for him too, growing closer means full honesty. I agree with you about that as well. (Criterion 1) From his position, what type of response would you expect if you were to say, **"Honesty and trust is really important to me—especially in our relationship. I have something I need to tell you: 10 years ago I gave up my child for adoption because I was using drugs at the time and couldn't be a good parent."** (Criterion 2)

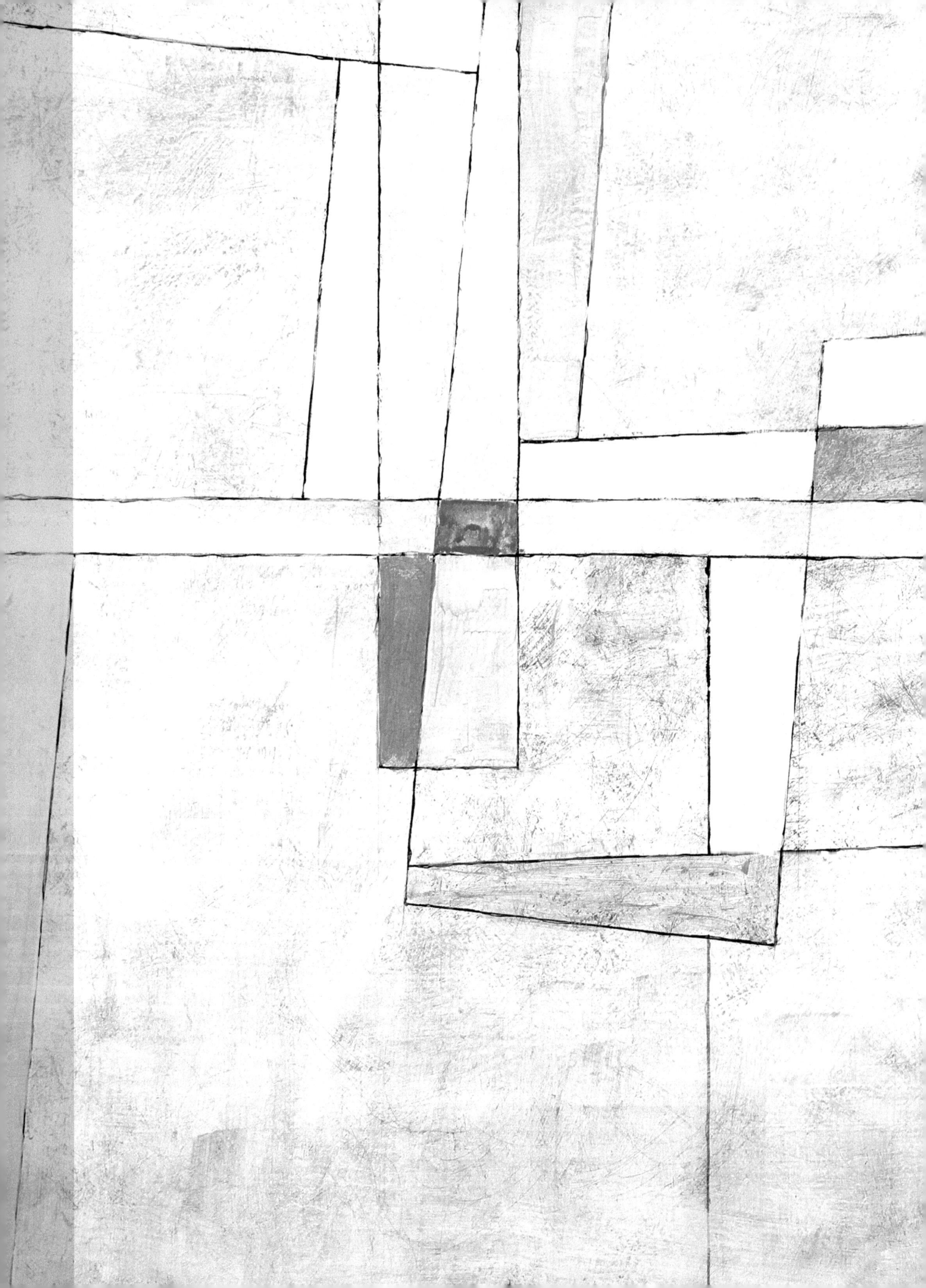

Mobilizing Social Support

Preparations for Exercise 9

1. Read the instructions in Chapter 2.

2. Download the Deliberate Practice Reaction Form and the Deliberate Practice Diary Form at https://www.apa.org/pubs/books/deliberate-practice-interpersonal-psychotherapy (see the "Resources" tab; also available in Appendixes A and B, respectively).

Skill Description

Skill Difficulty Level: Advanced

Interpersonal psychotherapy (IPT) helps clients strengthen social support as a way of reducing distress. To do this, the therapist works with clients to identify their support needs and then better connect with people in their life to receive the needed support. Improved social support is a change mechanism in IPT. The Interpersonal Inventory (Exercises 1 and 2) is often a good place to start to identify people who can support the client.

The mobilizing social support skill is designed to engage individuals in the client's support network for a clear and specific purpose across any of the four categories of commonly identified social support (emotional, instrumental, informational, or self-appraisal). Because clients in distress often have a difficult time recognizing their support needs or reaching out to others, the purpose of this skill is to assist clients in clearly identifying their need and then actively engaging their social network to access the support they need.

Mobilizing social support should generate client action. This move-to-action goal makes it a bit more difficult and is similar to the end goal of communication analysis and

https://doi.org/10.1037/0000426-011

Deliberate Practice in Interpersonal Psychotherapy, by O. Belik, J. M. Schultz, S. Fairhurst, S. Stuart, A. Vaz, and T. Rousmaniere

generating communication options. Next, Exercise 10, "Motivating Interpersonal Action," ties all of these skills together.

These advanced skills follow the previous IPT skills, which seek to promote insight or emotional awareness (e.g., interpersonal framing of distress and helping the client to describe their distress and need for support). These different skills complement one another to facilitate both greater interpersonal awareness and more effective interpersonal actions.

The therapist should improvise a response to each client statement following these skill criteria:

1. **Collaboratively clarify the client's interpersonal support need(s).** Clarifying and collaboratively understanding specific need for support is the first critical step in this skill because it explicitly defines and normalizes the need for help and support. This builds on the skills of clarification and helping the client to describe their distress and need for support. The goal is for the therapist to move the client to action in concrete ways. A typical prompt is: "Based on what we have been discussing and you have described, it seems to me that you really need some practical help with child care and some emotional support too—someone to recognize how difficult this has been for you. Do I have that right?"

2. **Direct the client to identify specific people in their social support network to meet their need(s).** After the need is collaboratively clarified, the therapist moves the client to activate their support network by compassionately highlighting the opportunity to engage others to get the support needed. In this circumstance, a *directive* can be understood as anything the therapist does to increase the likelihood of change. For instance, the directive might take the form of a homework assignment to have a conversation with another individual to ask for support. A less direct intervention might be to speculate with the client about how a request for help from another person on their Circle might go and how that might meet their needs. Even less direct but still effective could be to ask the client what ideas they have about asking another specific individual for support. In all cases, the clinician is moving the client toward action.

   A typical prompt is: "It sounds like your partner could help in meeting your needs, both the practical support with child care and the emotional support you need. I am thinking a direct conversation with him about what you need and why would be really helpful. When could you do that?"

SKILL CRITERIA FOR EXERCISE 9

1. Collaboratively clarify the client's interpersonal support need(s).
2. Direct the client to identify specific people in their social support network to meet their need(s).

Examples of Therapists Mobilizing Social Support

Example 1

CLIENT: [*motivated*] I feel like I need to get to the gym and get more exercise.

THERAPIST: That's great that you're wanting to be more active! Many people I've worked with find it really helpful to exercise with someone else—it makes them more likely to actually get to the gym. (Criterion 1) Who can you ask to go to the gym with you? (Criterion 2)

Example 2

CLIENT: [*frustrated*] My friend asked me to go to a concert this weekend, but I've got to stay home with the kids.

THERAPIST: It sounds like you need some help with child care so you can have some time to connect with your friend. (Criterion 1) Who can you ask to watch the kids and when could you ask them? (Criterion 2)

Example 3

CLIENT: [*angry*] I'm drowning in this huge project at work and I don't know if I can do this much longer.

THERAPIST: It sounds like you may need some help with this big project so it doesn't crush you. (Criterion 1) What kind of help or support could your coworkers give on this project, and how would you ask them for it? (Criterion 2)

INSTRUCTIONS FOR EXERCISE 9

Step 1: Role-Play and Feedback

- The client says the first beginner client statement. The therapist **improvises** a response based on the skill criteria.
- The trainer (or, if not available, the client) provides **brief** feedback based on the skill criteria.
- The client then repeats the same statement, and the therapist again improvises a response. The trainer (or client) again provides brief feedback.

Step 2: Repeat

- Repeat Step 1 for all the statements **in the current difficulty level** (beginner, intermediate, or advanced).

Step 3: Assess and Adjust Difficulty

- The therapist completes the Deliberate Practice Reaction Form (see Appendix A) and decides whether to make the exercise easier or harder or to repeat the same difficulty level.

Step 4: Repeat for Approximately 15 Minutes

- Repeat Steps 1 to 3 for at least 15 minutes.
- The trainees then switch therapist and client roles and start over.

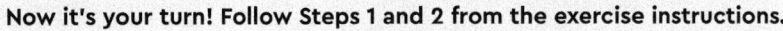

Now it's your turn! Follow Steps 1 and 2 from the exercise instructions.

Remember: The goal of the role-play is for trainees to practice improvising responses to the client statements in a manner that (a) uses the skill criteria and (b) feels authentic for the trainee. **Example therapist responses for each client statement are provided at the end of this exercise. Trainees should attempt to improvise their own responses before reading the examples.**

BEGINNER-LEVEL CLIENT STATEMENTS FOR EXERCISE 9
Beginner Client Statement 1
[Sad] I know I need to clean out my dad's house. He's been gone for 6 months now. But I'm dreading sorting through all his stuff by myself.
Beginner Client Statement 2
[Exacerbated] The bills just keep coming. I don't even know where to start. How am I ever going to get out of this mess of debt?
Beginner Client Statement 3
[Frustrated] What's the point anyway? I'm just going to fail this next test like I've failed the others because I'm a failure and I'm terrible at tests.
Beginner Client Statement 4
[Overwhelmed] I know it would be so much better for my family if we ate better, and I'd feel better too. I just don't have the time. I'm a single mom, there's only so much I can do.
Beginner Client Statement 5
[Dejected] I wish I could go to college. I have no idea if it's even possible or how I could make it work since I'm undocumented.

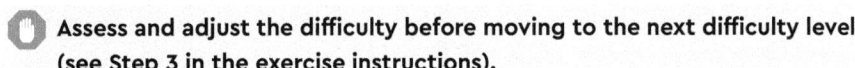 **Assess and adjust the difficulty before moving to the next difficulty level (see Step 3 in the exercise instructions).**

INTERMEDIATE-LEVEL CLIENT STATEMENTS FOR EXERCISE 9
Intermediate Client Statement 1
[Sad] This house is just so empty without my partner.
Intermediate Client Statement 2
[Anxious] I don't want to miss my daughter's wedding, but I'm so scared to travel. I don't know if I can do it.
Intermediate Client Statement 3
[Confused] I'm so overwhelmed with what's happening with my son's chemo treatments. The doctors and the nurses seem to be saying different things about what he needs and what I should be doing. My son keeps asking me questions, and he sees that I'm scared. I don't know what to tell him.
Intermediate Client Statement 4
[Deflated] When I try to talk to my husband about everything that's happening, he tries to fix it. I just want him to listen.
Intermediate Client Statement 5
[Overwhelmed] It's my duty as the oldest to take care of my dad now, and I want to do it, I really do. But I'm just so overwhelmed by it all—the doctor's appointments, the medications. . . . Trying to be sure he's okay when I've also got to take care of my own kids and life.

✋ **Assess and adjust the difficulty before moving to the next difficulty level (see Step 3 in the exercise instructions).**

ADVANCED CLIENT STATEMENTS FOR EXERCISE 9
Advanced Client Statement 1
[Depressed] I just can't get out of bed. I'm going to lose my job . . . I just know it.
Advanced Client Statement 2
[Sad] I just barely failed the vision test, and they took away my driver's license. What am I going to do? My independence is gone.
Advanced Client Statement 3
[Hopeless] No one understands what it's like to have a child with an addiction because they've never had to deal with it. I feel so alone.
Advanced Client Statement 4
[Longingly] I miss my family back in Guatemala. I don't want them to worry about me, but I just miss them.
Advanced Client Statement 5
[Angry] I don't understand how people can just go on like nothing's happening. We're destroying the planet, and I feel like I am the only one who cares.

Assess and adjust the difficulty here (see Step 3 in the exercise instructions). If appropriate, follow the instructions to make the exercise even more challenging (see Appendix A).

Example Therapist Responses: Mobilizing Social Support

Remember: Trainees should attempt to improvise their own responses before reading the example responses. **Do not read the following responses verbatim unless you are having trouble coming up with your own!**

EXAMPLE RESPONSES TO BEGINNER-LEVEL CLIENT STATEMENTS FOR EXERCISE 9
Example Response to Beginner Client Statement 1
It sounds like you need some help to start this enormous task of sorting through your dad's home. (Criterion 1) Who could you ask to help you with that? (Criterion 2)
Example Response to Beginner Client Statement 2
It sounds like you need some practical help in figuring out where to start. (Criterion 1) Who might be able to help you make a plan to tackle this debt? (Criterion 2)
Example Response to Beginner Client Statement 3
We all need a little help at times, especially when things are challenging. It sounds like this may be one of those times. Sounds like you need some practical help in studying for the next test and someone to help build your confidence too. (Criterion 1) I wonder who on your Interpersonal Circle might be able to help you prepare for it—could that same person help with your confidence too? How would you ask them for that? (Criterion 2)
Example Response to Beginner Client Statement 4
I hear you saying better nutrition is important for you and your family's health, and you need some practical help to make that happen. (Criterion 1) Who can help you with things like choosing foods, or grocery shopping, or meal prep, or other things that take time, and how do you imagine asking them to help you? (Criterion 2)
Example Response to Beginner Client Statement 5
It sounds like you need some help to understand what your rights and options for college are. (Criterion 1) Who can you trust with the information about your status that might also be able to help you in learning about what is possible for the future? (Criterion 2)

EXAMPLE RESPONSES TO INTERMEDIATE-LEVEL CLIENT STATEMENTS FOR EXERCISE 9
Example Response to Intermediate Client Statement 1
It sounds like you are lonely and need to be around other people as you are dealing with this relationship loss. (Criterion 1). Is there someone on your Interpersonal Circle that you can reach out to who you could spend time with this week, and what would you want to do with them? (Criterion 2)
Example Response to Intermediate Client Statement 2
Being there for your daughter is really important to you. I think that anyone would feel the same way. It sounds like you need some direct support in navigating the travel to the wedding—someone to fly with you who will be able to reassure you and help you stay calm. (Criterion 1) Let's look at your Interpersonal Circle and think through who could come with you as a support and provide the reassurance you need. (Criterion 2)
Example Response to Intermediate Client Statement 3
I'm so sorry this is happening. Anyone in your situation would be struggling. The medical system is so complex that it is hard to get information and to understand what is going on. It sounds like you need some more information and clarity on your son's needs from his health care team. (Criterion 1) Who specifically can help get you that information, and how can you ask them for their help? (Criterion 2)
Example Response to Intermediate Client Statement 4
It sounds like you need your husband to recognize that he can better support you by just listening to you. Sometimes other people don't realize this unless you tell them directly. (Criterion 1) How can you help him understand the kind of support you need, and when could you have that conversation with him? (Criterion 2)
Example Response to Intermediate Client Statement 5
With all that is on your plate, it makes sense that you need some help in managing things. (Criterion 1) Who could you ask to help you occasionally with caring for your dad or your kids? (Criterion 2)

EXAMPLE RESPONSES TO ADVANCED-LEVEL CLIENT STATEMENTS FOR EXERCISE 9
Example Response to Advanced Client Statement 1
Given all you are dealing with, it's understandable that you need help to get your daily activities done. (Criterion 1) Who can you ask to help you get out of bed in the morning and get to work? What specifically do you want them to do? (Criterion 2)
Example Response to Advanced Client Statement 2
This would be a big transition for anyone. It sounds like you're going to need some practical help in getting to where you want to go, but I also think I hear a need for some understanding from others about what this is like for you. (Criterion 1) How might you find people that could help you with transportation and rides? Who do you think could really understand what this is like for you? (Criterion 2)
Example Response to Advanced Client Statement 3
It sounds like it would be really helpful for you to connect with other parents who get what it's like to have a child with an addiction. (Criterion 1) I'd like to suggest that you try going to the Al-Anon group here in town. That group is for parents who have family members with addiction, and I have worked with many parents who found it helpful. What do you think about going to a group meeting to try it out? (Criterion 2)
Example Response to Advanced Client Statement 4
Of course you miss them, they are so very important to you. I imagine they miss you too. It sounds like you need to find more ways to stay connected to your family. (Criterion 1) I wonder if you might be able to schedule more opportunities to call them? (Criterion 2)
Example Response to Advanced Client Statement 5
I wonder if it would be helpful to connect with others who share your deep concern for our planet. (Criterion 1) We could spend a few minutes right now in session looking up groups that are trying to support pro-ecology causes. Would you be willing to try one of those groups? (Criterion 2)

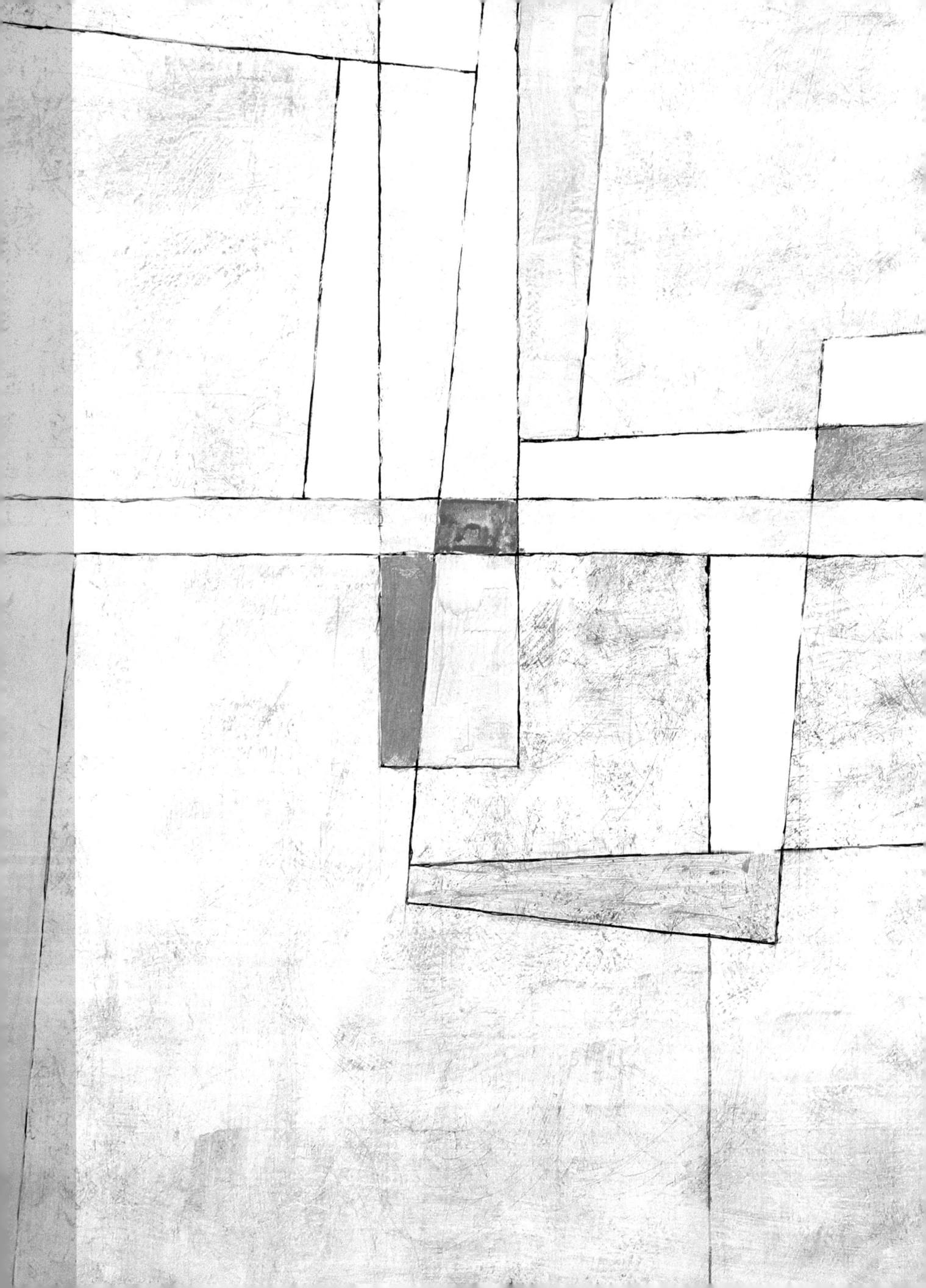

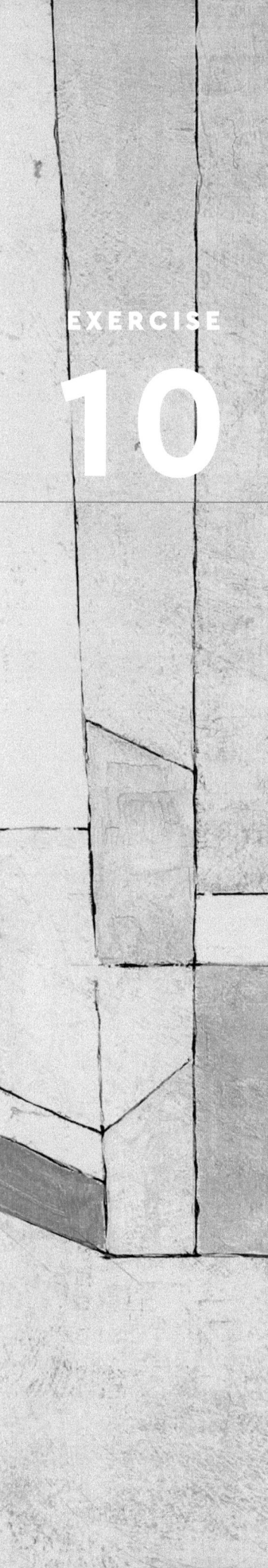

Motivating Interpersonal Action

Preparations for Exercise 10

1. Read the instructions in Chapter 2.

2. Download the Deliberate Practice Reaction Form and the Deliberate Practice Diary Form at https://www.apa.org/pubs/books/deliberate-practice-interpersonal-psychotherapy (see the "Resources" tab; also available in Appendixes A and B, respectively).

Skill Description

Skill Difficulty Level: Advanced

The goal of this skill is to encourage clients to engage their Interpersonal Circle, and address clients' reluctance for doing so. Taking interpersonal action to address an unhealthy relationship or to change communication with others requires a belief that the efforts might actually change things. With depression, however, there is an insidious tendency for people to isolate themselves. This tendency can be rooted in any number of experiences, from anhedonia ("I just don't want to do anything anymore"), to decreased appetite ("Why would I go to a restaurant—I don't feel like eating anyway"), to decreased energy ("Going to the meeting feels like so much more than I can do"), to feeling like a burden ("I just tend to bring everyone else down—I'll just stay at home").

The client's real lived experience with relationships, including times that other people may have been unhelpful or maybe even damaging, may understandably lead them to be skeptical that other people will respond in a helpful and healthy way. Motivation to engage one's social network requires the client to feel self-efficacious that they are able to make the attempts, as well as a belief that their social network is likely to respond more positively. An interpersonal psychotherapy therapist has to have a strategy to motivate and inspire the client to action.

https://doi.org/10.1037/0000426-012

Deliberate Practice in Interpersonal Psychotherapy, by O. Belik, J. M. Schultz, S. Fairhurst, S. Stuart, A. Vaz, and T. Rousmaniere

The therapist should improvise a response to each client statement following these skill criteria:

1. **Reflect and enhance the client's readiness to engage in a new interpersonal action.** In-session role-playing is designed to increase the client's skills and confidence that they are ready to engage with their support network in a healthy way. In this skill, the therapist starts by conveying their belief that the client is now ready to try engaging in a new interpersonal action. This is achieved by commenting on the growth of the client's skills and confidence, or enthusiastically agreeing with the client's decision to engage in said new action.

2. **Encourage a specific interpersonal action the client can implement.** To build a pattern of success, there is wisdom in matching recommendations to the likelihood of success. For clients who may have less confidence in themselves and their support network, the therapist—in a posture of support and reassurance—should recommend an action that is less emotionally intense and that engages someone in the social network who is more likely to respond positively. Start with the easy tasks—the "low-hanging fruit."

   For clients who present more skeptically, recommendations can be more specific and limited, giving reason for hope for change with more manageable interpersonal risks. When the client's abilities are apparent and there are healthy members of the support network who are likely to respond well, the clinician can encourage more risk-taking.

SKILL CRITERIA FOR EXERCISE 10
1. Reflect and enhance the client's readiness to engage in a new interpersonal action. 2. Encourage a specific interpersonal action the client can implement.

Examples of Therapists Motivating Interpersonal Action

Example 1

CLIENT: [*optimistically*] I think I just might be able to ask the nurses for more help.

THERAPIST: I've observed your communication skills and you really are ready! (Criterion 1) Try it! I'll bet the nurses will respond well. (Criterion 2)

Example 2

CLIENT: [*skeptically*] Practicing with you feels easy but I worry that my boss will just roll her eyes when I ask for the time off I need.

THERAPIST: It feels easy because you're getting good at it. (Criterion 1) Maybe you can practice the first try with a colleague, to get a win before talking with your boss. (Criterion 2)

Example 3

CLIENT: [*dejected*] Without you there, being nice all the time, I don't think I can actually do it.

THERAPIST: I hear you, having the confidence to communicate well is a work in progress—and you're getting there. (Criterion 1) Maybe we could practice together with your husband during a session. (Criterion 2)

INSTRUCTIONS FOR EXERCISE 10

Step 1: Role-Play and Feedback

- The client says the first beginner client statement. The therapist **improvises** a response based on the skill criteria.
- The trainer (or, if not available, the client) provides **brief** feedback based on the skill criteria.
- The client then repeats the same statement, and the therapist again improvises a response. The trainer (or client) again provides brief feedback.

Step 2: Repeat

- Repeat Step 1 for all the statements **in the current difficulty level** (beginner, intermediate, or advanced).

Step 3: Assess and Adjust Difficulty

- The therapist completes the Deliberate Practice Reaction Form (see Appendix A) and decides whether to make the exercise easier or harder or to repeat the same difficulty level.

Step 4: Repeat for Approximately 15 Minutes

- Repeat Steps 1 to 3 for at least 15 minutes.
- The trainees then switch therapist and client roles and start over.

→ Now it's your turn! Follow Steps 1 and 2 from the instructions.

Remember: The goal of the role-play is for trainees to practice improvising responses to the client statements in a manner that (a) uses the skill criteria and (b) feels authentic for the trainee. **Example therapist responses for each client statement are provided at the end of this exercise. Trainees should attempt to improvise their own responses before reading the examples.**

BEGINNER-LEVEL CLIENT STATEMENTS FOR EXERCISE 10
Beginner Client Statement 1
[Hopeful] Taking a walk around the lake with my neighbor feels like something that would help.
Beginner Client Statement 2
[Confident] If I ask my daughter out to dinner, I bet we can start to reconnect.
Beginner Client Statement 3
[Appreciative] I think I'll take my brother up on his offer to help with the clutter in my apartment.
Beginner Client Statement 4
[Optimistic] I'm feeling less burned out, and I think I'm ready to show up to the employee wellness activity.
Beginner Client Statement 5
[Proud] I can be useful by offering to babysit my granddaughter.

 Assess and adjust the difficulty before moving to the next difficulty level (see Step 3 in the exercise instructions).

INTERMEDIATE-LEVEL CLIENT STATEMENTS FOR EXERCISE 10
Intermediate Client Statement 1
[Worried] I don't know how the others will react, but I'm ready to tell people about getting arrested.
Intermediate Client Statement 2
[Appreciative] I think I'm ready to rejoin the group. I'm still not sure if I can be fun to be around, but they're all nice and will probably include me either way.
Intermediate Client Statement 3
[Concerned] When he visits me this weekend I'll try to apologize. Let's hope he's in a good place.
Intermediate Client Statement 4
[Nervous] I haven't reached out to my old friend in over a decade. It will stun him when I send a text, but maybe he'll want to meet for drinks.
Intermediate Client Statement 5
[Resigned] After our role-plays, I think I've gotten over being sensitive. I'm going to join the conversation even if she rolls her eyes.

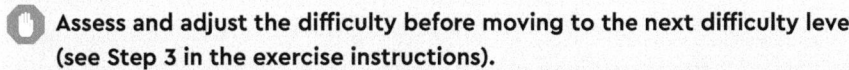 **Assess and adjust the difficulty before moving to the next difficulty level (see Step 3 in the exercise instructions).**

ADVANCED-LEVEL CLIENT STATEMENTS FOR EXERCISE 10
Advanced Client Statement 1
[Hopeless] I'm not sure if I'm ready to talk with her. It's just that I always seem to say the wrong thing and she always takes it as an insult.
Advanced Client Statement 2
[Resigned] I'm worried about my upcoming meeting with my boss. Every Zoom meeting, I can feel his contempt for me, no matter what I say.
Advanced Client Statement 3
[Discouraged] I have a job interview in 2 weeks but looking confident is really hard after five failed interviews.
Advanced Client Statement 4
[Withdrawn] I have been avoiding the supermarket because my ex-wife shops there a lot. I appreciate the help you have given me in communicating with her, but watch me still duck to the next aisle if I see her.
Advanced Client Statement 5
[Shaken] Despite our role-plays, I am still very nervous about talking with my brother about how he hasn't been paying his share of the rent. When the moment comes, I'll probably give in just to avoid another conflict.

 Assess and adjust the difficulty here (see Step 3 in the exercise instructions). If appropriate, follow the instructions to make the exercise even more challenging (see Appendix A).

Example Therapist Responses: Motivating Interpersonal Action

Remember: Trainees should attempt to improvise their own responses before reading the example responses. **Do not read the following responses verbatim unless you are having trouble coming up with your own!**

EXAMPLE RESPONSES TO BEGINNER-LEVEL CLIENT STATEMENTS FOR EXERCISE 10
Example Response to Beginner Client Statement 1
It sounds like you're ready to make that call and set up the walk. (Criterion 1) I can't wait to hear how they respond! (Criterion 2)
Example Response to Beginner Client Statement 2
I can really feel your desire to reconnect. (Criterion 1) Dinner will be a great chance to let her know how much you care. (Criterion 2)
Example Response to Beginner Client Statement 3
Great decision! (Criterion 1) I know you'll be able to let him know what you need. (Criterion 2)
Example Response to Beginner Client Statement 4
Burnout can get anyone, but it seems like you're ready to reengage now. (Criterion 1) You might really connect with a colleague or two. (Criterion 2)
Example Response to Beginner Client Statement 5
I love how helping others is helpful to you. Caring for others is a great way to start feeling better—to give meaning to your life. (Criterion 1) Make that offer, and I'll bet they take you up on it. (Criterion 2)

EXAMPLE RESPONSES TO INTERMEDIATE-LEVEL CLIENT STATEMENTS FOR EXERCISE 10
Example Response to Intermediate Client Statement 1
I'm impressed that you're ready to be open. (Criterion 1) Who, in the group, feels like the best person to start with? (Criterion 2)
Example Response to Intermediate Client Statement 2
Your willingness to rejoin is great. (Criterion 1) Having such an accepting group means it's okay for you to be there without pressure to be the life of the party. (Criterion 2)
Example Response to Intermediate Client Statement 3
We've practiced and I know you're ready. (Criterion 1) Let's identify signals to look for to spot when he's in a good place so you can maximize the chance that the conversation goes well. (Criterion 2)
Example Response to Intermediate Client Statement 4
You're ready to send it and to respond to his reaction. I'm confident that this is the case since we've practiced and thought through what to send in the text. (Criterion 1) Setting up the get-together is something we can celebrate—a great first step. (Criterion 2)
Example Response to Intermediate Client Statement 5
Exactly, our role-plays have helped you get ready. (Criterion 1) You can join the conversation and stay composed, even if there are eyerolls. (Criterion 2)

EXAMPLE RESPONSES TO ADVANCED-LEVEL
CLIENT STATEMENTS FOR EXERCISE 10

Example Response to Advanced Client Statement 1

You've worked hard in our practice together, but I can understand it's still hard to feel confident putting practice into action. (Criterion 1) This is a first step, so you don't have to go into anything deep at all. (Criterion 2)

Example Response to Advanced Client Statement 2

In our role-plays, you've done a great job of keeping the tone positive. (Criterion 1) It's still hard, he may take a while to come around, but you can start with simply being on the call and making a comment or two to show you are present and participating. (Criterion 2)

Example Response to Advanced Client Statement 3

The rejections are discouraging, that's for sure. Even if you're skeptical right now, you've come across as more self-assured in our mock interviews. (Criterion 1) I'm confident you will come across that way this time too. The practice will pay off. (Criterion 2)

Example Response to Advanced Client Statement 4

You've made a lot of progress practicing positive communication with her in our role-plays. (Criterion 1) I think you will do great if you believe in yourself and stay positive, just like we practiced. (Criterion 2)

Example Response to Advanced Client Statement 5

It's true that our role-plays don't have the same pressure that you're going to feel in real-life moments. But you've practiced, and you've already improved. (Criterion 1) Now it's time to put that into action. I'll look forward to hearing how it goes. (Criterion 2)

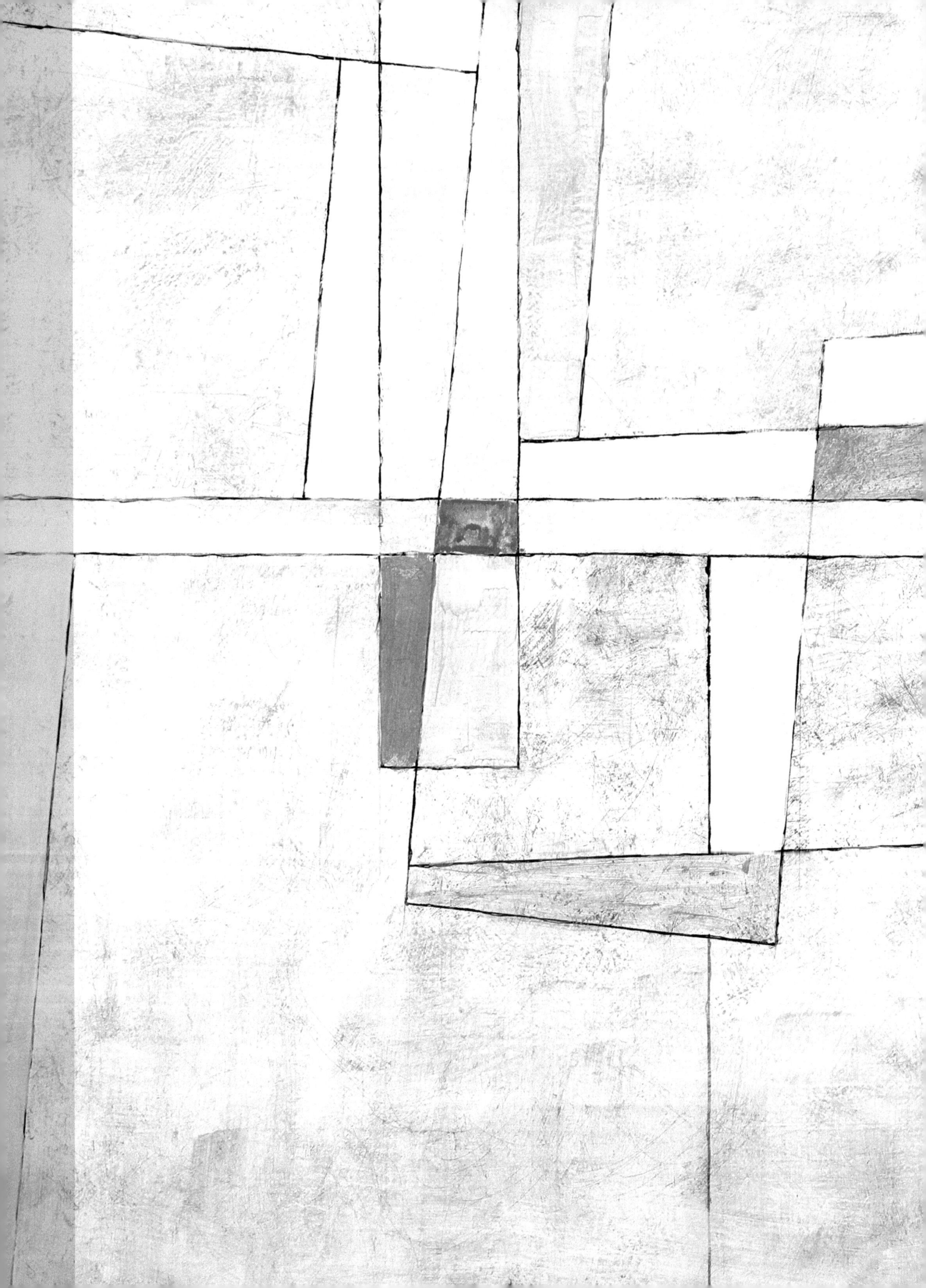

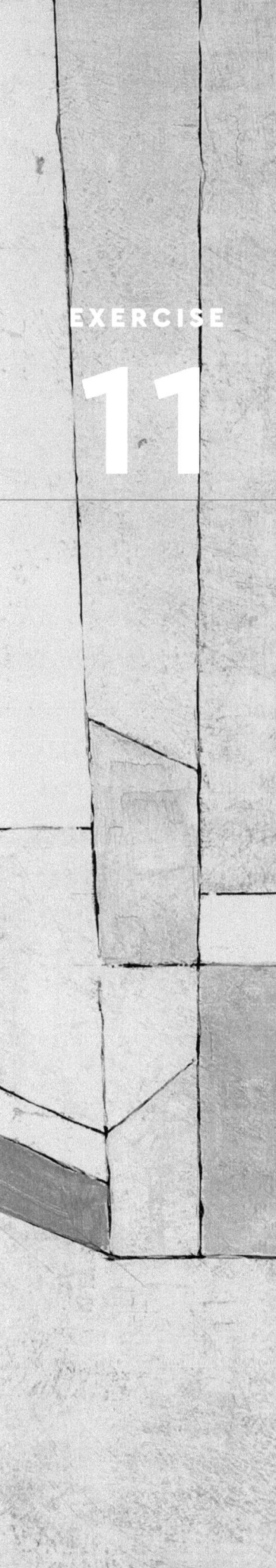

Annotated Interpersonal Psychotherapy Practice Session Transcript

Now you get a chance to put all the skills you have learned together! This exercise is a transcript of a session that is condensed to include aspects of each of the 10 skills you have learned. Each skill is labeled, providing an example of how therapists can include skills that are responsive to client needs.

Instructions

One trainee can play the therapist while the other plays the client, displaying a tone and affect congruent with the material. Both participants can read line-by-line from the transcript. As with all deliberate practice, try it again! The purpose of this transcript is to provide you with an opportunity to experience how it feels to offer all the interpersonal psychotherapy skills in the context of a session, albeit condensed, yet one that mimics live therapy.

Annotated Interpersonal Psychotherapy Transcript

THERAPIST 1: So, what I'd like to do in this session is what I call an Interpersonal Inventory with you. An Interpersonal Inventory is a summary or a picture representing your social support network. Would that be okay with you? (Skill 1: Presenting the Interpersonal Inventory, present the plan for the session to conduct an Interpersonal Inventory)

CLIENT 1: It's been changing lately, so it will probably be good for me to understand it better.

THERAPIST 2: Great. It will help both of us to gain a better understanding about what your social network looks like, the kinds of support you're getting, and why some of the relationships are a bit more difficult for you. (Skill 1: Presenting the Interpersonal Inventory, present a rationale for the use of the Interpersonal Inventory)

https://doi.org/10.1037/0000426-013

Deliberate Practice in Interpersonal Psychotherapy, by O. Belik, J. M. Schultz, S. Fairhurst, S. Stuart, A. Vaz, and T. Rousmaniere

CLIENT 2: [*nods*] Yes, that would help me.

THERAPIST 3: So what I'd like you to do is to take a piece of paper and try to draw two big circles, one big one, and then another one inside it—kind of like a donut or a bagel is one way to picture it. (Skill 1: Presenting the Interpersonal Inventory)

CLIENT 3: Got it. [*draws circles on paper*] Okay.

THERAPIST 4: And could you hold that up to the screen so I could see what you've got?

CLIENT 4: [*holds up paper with circles*] Here it is.

THERAPIST 5: Perfect. So what I'd like you to do is to imagine that you're in the middle of the Circle and to write down the names of the seven to 10 people, maybe more, depending on how close they are to you and the kind of support you're getting from them. In the inner circle, you can put your "intimate" supports—people who provide you with a great deal of support. The one right outside of that could include your "close support" people, those who are important but not quite so close or supportive, and the rest of the space would include your "extended" supports, people who are a bit further away from you. Sometimes people put individuals who passed away some time ago and are still important to them on the Circle. Some people put pets on the Circle as well. There are no right or wrong choices, and you can include anyone you'd like. What I am interested in is your perspective. (Skill 1: Presenting the Interpersonal Inventory)

CLIENT 5: Okay, I think I understand.

THERAPIST 6: So, do you have any questions about what I'm looking for there? (Skill 1: Presenting the Interpersonal Inventory)

CLIENT 6: No, I think I've got it. Umm, can you say it again? You're looking for like seven to 10 people?

THERAPIST 7: Could be more or less than that, whatever feels right to you.

CLIENT 7: OK, got it. [*client writes names in the circles*]

THERAPIST 8: Okay, excellent. Could you hold that up so I can see it?

CLIENT 8: Yeah, here it is.

THERAPIST 9: Excellent. We'll make a copy of that too, so we can both use it as we move forward in therapy together. (Skill 2: Exploring Interpersonal Relationships)

CLIENT 9: Sounds good.

THERAPIST 10: That's really helpful to see it, the visual representation of your support. I hope it's helpful for you too. Now what I'd like to do is to find out about each of those relationships in some detail. Who would you like to introduce me to first? (Skill 2: Exploring Interpersonal Relationships)

CLIENT 10: Yes, this is helpful for me too. You know, there are two people who are kind of moving in opposite directions right now.

THERAPIST 11: [*empathically*] I see, can you tell me more about the two people?

CLIENT 11: My wife and I are separated, so she's kind of moving from the inner circle toward the outer one, and my mom found out that she has Stage 4 cancer. And we have always been close, but now it feels like she's closer than ever.

THERAPIST 12: That's gotta be really difficult for you, that kind of disconnection from your wife, and I'm sorry to hear about your mom's cancer diagnosis; that must be difficult as well.

CLIENT 12: Uh, thanks. Yeah, it's, it's really disorienting . . .

THERAPIST 13: I hear you. It does sound like there are some relational changes happening right now. So, who would you like to start with first?

CLIENT 13: Maybe I will start with my mom.

THERAPIST 14: Could you tell me about what that relationship is like? (Skill 2: Exploring Interpersonal Relationships)

CLIENT 14: You know, we've always been close, and she loves my kids, and you know, it's a big family. I have three kids, but then my brother and sister each have kids of their own. But even though visiting our house is like a little elementary school, it's like every time I see my mom, she somehow is able to bring the energy.

THERAPIST 15: Sounds like your mom has incredible energy. And now, you mentioned the cancer diagnosis.

CLIENT 15: And she decided not to get chemo. Uh. Yeah, I—I can't imagine not having her around, and it's hard for me to think of anything else.

THERAPIST 16: Yeah. I can only imagine what you're all going through.

CLIENT 16: Yeah. Not easy.

THERAPIST 17: What are the aspects about the relationship that you feel are really supportive? (Skill 2: Exploring Interpersonal Relationships, practice using different questions)

CLIENT 17: Like me supporting her?

THERAPIST 18: Good question. Let's start with support coming from her. We will talk about your support for her in just a moment. What kind of support do you get from her? (Skill 2: Exploring the Interpersonal Inventory, practice using different questions)

CLIENT 18: You know, lately it's been the way that she supports helping raise my kids, especially since now I'm doing that part of the week on my own with the separation. She comes over to the house at least twice a week just to help out and be a presence, and it's like she, yeah, supports without asking anything in return.

THERAPIST 19: Well, that's even more remarkable. Given that she's going through cancer and still is able to do that for you.

CLIENT 19: Exactly.

THERAPIST 20: How would you say that you support her? (Skill 2: Exploring Interpersonal Relationships, practice using different questions)

CLIENT 20: You know. I try to be supportive, but it's so frustrating that she won't—she won't get the treatment. I mean, I acknowledge it's her right not to get it. And I've told her so and that I can't change her mind about that. Umm. And I know it wouldn't help anything for me to—to be angry or even try to talk her out of it. So I try to support by just telling her, you know, it's her right and I respect that.

THERAPIST 21: You've done a great job of describing how supportive she is and some of the frustrations that you experience supporting her. How would you like the relationship to be different? (Skill 3: Clarifications, briefly and accurately summarize client's statement)

CLIENT 21: You know now that it's temporary in nature. It's odd for me to even put those words out there. I want her to understand how much I appreciate her and how much I sort of owe her.

THERAPIST 22: [*empathically*] I see.

CLIENT 22: Uh, she wouldn't think of it that way, but I know I do.

THERAPIST 23: One of the things I have found really helpful is having people tell me a story about the person that we're talking about on the Interpersonal Inventory. It's another way of understanding what the relationship is like. What kind of story comes to mind for you about your mom? (Skill 2: Exploring Interpersonal Relationships, practice using different questions)

CLIENT 23: She was in the kitchen with the kids just last week and they were baking together. And of course, my sons are always trying to add extra sugar—extra brown sugar. Umm. And she's laughing and finding a way to make it all work. And next thing you know, I had some other work to do, so I left for a few, then I went back. And then I saw the four of them dancing to Taylor Swift while the cookies were in the oven. And I think, here's someone who's gotten the worst news they could possibly get and somehow she's just bringing joy.

THERAPIST 24: Hmm. Yeah, that's a great story, and I can imagine that'd be a wonderful one to hang on to, to commemorate. Some of the stories can be really helpful as you're going through grief and loss. So thanks for sharing that one.

CLIENT 24: Thanks for listening.

THERAPIST 25: Let's look at one of the other relationships you described—your relationship with your wife. It sounded like that one is moving apart. Can you help me understand that better? (Skill 2: Exploring Interpersonal Relationships, practice using different questions)

CLIENT 25: Maybe I don't fully understand it, but I can kind of tell you. What she says is that since I'm kind of feeling frustrated and hopeless about work and about, you know, not having the friends I used to have, she said it was just exhausting to be around me and she needed a break. And I know I'm not the only one going through stuff, but I don't know if the break is permanent or not. And I guess it's not really up to me to decide. But yeah, I don't see how taking a guy whose career has stalled and his mom has cancer . . . I don't see how taking a break helps, but here we are.

THERAPIST 26: Yeah, so if I hear you correctly, somehow she's communicating to you that you're a burden to her in some way or that she can't manage what you're going through. Can you help me understand that better? (Skill 3: Clarifications, briefly and accurately summarize the client's statement, ask the client a question that helps them further describe their experience)

CLIENT 26: I mean what she said to me was, "I don't know what you should do." That's the quote I keep hearing. But she felt she needed to take care of herself because she was just, with me, not in a place that was bringing her any kind of joy.

THERAPIST 27: I hear you say she did not feel joy with you. When you say "joy," what do you understand she means? Can you say more about it? (Skill 3: Clarifications, briefly and accurately summarize the client's statement, ask the client a question that helps them to describe their experience further)

CLIENT 27: Fun, relief, or anything like that. And, and I, I get it. Umm. You know, even when I came back and saw my mom dancing to Taylor Swift with the kids, part of it was that I had to, you know, step away to catch up on some work. But I wasn't really able to catch up on work. I was just thinking about how things aren't working out.

THERAPIST 28: Yeah. I think I'm hearing between the lines—and please correct me if I'm off here—but I think I'm hearing that this is not what you want but that the decision to leave is hers. Am I on track there? (Skill **4:** Interpersonal Framing of Distress, reflect the client's distress)

CLIENT 28: That's exactly right. I wasn't really surprised when she decided to leave. Umm, but it's not what I wanted at all. I'm not mad, I guess I can't blame her, though. I get it, I guess.

THERAPIST 29: Yeah. Where you said about not feeling mad, but one of the things I'm wondering is, what kinds of emotional reactions you're having. But I think I might be hearing a sense of being abandoned, but I don't think that is quite the right word. So could you help me understand better about what that's like and what words you would use to describe it? (Skill 4: Interpersonal Framing of Distress, connect the client's distress with interpersonal issues they are experiencing)

CLIENT 29: You know, if I were to think of my wife and my mom as two major supportive people, and like all of a sudden instead of two steady and strong people, it's like one's got cracks and is crumbling and the other took off. So yeah. I think I feel, uh, weird and at the same time, kind of hopeless and kind of scared.

THERAPIST 30: Yeah, that's a really helpful description of things. Especially how you described one having cracks and one that took off. It puts it in such simple language that's easy to understand, but the hopelessness and stress that you're describing really comes through clearly. And it sounds like that—like that's directly related to the upcoming loss of your mom. And if I can be so direct, the loss of relationship support from your wife at the same time, at least for right now. Do I have that right? (Skill 4: Interpersonal Framing of Distress, check to determine if this potential connection makes sense to the client)

CLIENT 30: No, you got it. Either one on its own would have knocked me down, but both at once seems to have—I don't even know.

THERAPIST 31: I had somebody describe it to me one time in a certain way, and I want to check and make sure this makes sense to you. This person said it's as if that sense of hopelessness, of feeling overwhelmed is like standing on a beach and a huge tidal wave comes in and knocks you over. (Skill 5: Helping the Client Describe Their Distress and Need for Support, summarize the emotional needs of the client)

CLIENT 31: That's it.

THERAPIST 32: Before you can even get up, another one comes in.

CLIENT 32: Meanwhile, each of those waves pulls the sand out from under my feet.

THERAPIST 33: Yeah, thanks for helping me understand that better. That was extremely helpful for me. I particularly liked that visual metaphor of the waves and the sand being pulled out from underneath your feet. So from an emotional standpoint, what kinds of support or understanding do you need? How would you describe that? (Skill 5: Helping the Client Describe Their Distress and Need for Support, prompt the client to explain specifically what the fulfillment of that need would look like in their relationships)

CLIENT 33: I wish I could just be tough enough on my own to let my mom know how much she means and how much I'll miss her, but I keep thinking about what it is that I'm going to miss and can't find a way to actually say it. What kind of support do I need for that?

THERAPIST 34: Right. So, when you do think about all the people in your life who can provide you with support now, who comes to mind?

CLIENT 34: My ex comes to mind. Maybe I do have to reach out to my ex. Also, I do have some friends at work and I've got some friends at the gym, but none of them are people that I talk to that closely. I guess, right now, I also have the support from you.

THERAPIST 35: That makes sense for now.

CLIENT 35: I'd like to be able to be in the kind of place where I could say the things that are helpful and meaningful to my mom, without my own hopelessness or my frustration becoming something that she has to take care of.

THERAPIST 36: Okay. Because one of the things we're doing in therapy is working on just increasing social support, generally including friends, some of the connections that you were describing. But one of the things we can also do is to practice here in session. How that conversation might go and what you want to get across. If I can ask you, what emotional support do you need to have that conversation with your mom? (Skill 5: Helping the Client Describe Their Distress and Need for Support, prompt the client to explain specifically what the fulfillment of that need would look like in their relationships)

CLIENT 36: I need someone to help me just recognize and say out loud that this . . . this is the end of someone's life.

THERAPIST 37: Who might be that someone? (Skill 9: Mobilizing Social Support)

CLIENT 37: Given her always being the one helping each of us, I'm not the only one going through this. I mean, now that you mention it, my brother and my sister—it's just, it's not like this is a foreign thing to them. They're going through something similar and maybe—maybe—they would be good people for me to talk to. My brother and I can actually talk pretty easily about this stuff, so maybe that could work. I mean, I really haven't thought about it, like having a deeper talk with them. I think I can do it.

THERAPIST 38: Now that you are thinking about it, it sounds like you can talk to them and are ready to do it. (Skill 10: Motivating Interpersonal Action)

CLIENT 38: Yes, maybe that would be smart to do . . .

THERAPIST 39: That was one of the things that struck me too, just thinking back to the Circle that you shared with me. The other people who are going through this too, who maybe could understand a lot more about what it's like. And I can imagine it being mutually supportive. If you were to do that.

CLIENT 39: It's funny that it hadn't even occurred to me until just now.

THERAPIST 40: So as we've been talking about this, one of the things that I think has been extremely helpful is the way you've described things so well. I feel like I understand a lot better what this kind of one–two punch the tidal wave is. That's such a helpful metaphor and helps to understand things well. I wonder what would happen if you used those terms in conversation with your brother. How do you think that might work? (Skill 6: Reinforcement of Effective Communication, identify the client's effective use of interpersonal communication in session, reinforce how this effective communication positively influences their ability to be understood by the therapist, suggest further use of effective communication strategy outside of session)

CLIENT 40: Yeah, you know, setting aside time that we could talk. That's doable. You know, he's always been easy to talk to and he's always been someone who likes to think on the bright side of things and doesn't want to dwell on the negative. But at the same time, I mean this is real and right in our face. This isn't about, like, who's got a negative outlook and who's bubbly. Umm, I think we could talk about what we'll miss with her, but also how to—how to be with her for the time that we've got left.

THERAPIST 41: Yeah, it seems like that would be extremely helpful to have that conversation. One of the things I'm curious about is, could you tell me about a recent time, or maybe the last time, that the two of you even touched on your mom's cancer diagnosis and what was happening? (Skill 7: Communication Analysis, ask the client for relevant details about a specific interpersonal incident)

CLIENT 41: Umm, you know, she had gone in to the doctor for a whole different reason. Uh, and then they had some suspicions and they did a scan or however they test, and she turns out to be Stage 4, no symptoms. My brother kept saying the tests are wrong. And then it switched to "Well, you know, there's stories about people who can live a long time with this." And I was trying to tell him, you know, no, this is this big. Meanwhile, I don't think she knows fully how much we care. And I know that when I talk to her, those words don't come out like they should, because I get upset that she's not doing what I consider to be fighting the cancer. So, it just comes out wrong—it's almost like I can't go there.

THERAPIST 42: Right. I think we're working toward communicating to your mom what you're experiencing. In this situation, it would be really helpful if you could tell me about the last time you and your mom interacted when you tried to or thought about sharing with her some of the feelings that you're having and how much she means to you. Can you tell me about the last time that happened? (Skill 7: Communication Analysis, ask the client for relevant details about a specific Interpersonal Incident)

CLIENT 42: You know, all of this is a fairly recent development. It's only been two months since we found out. Right after, uh, she found out, she spoke to my sister first and talked to me second. She had sworn to my sister not to say anything. I kept trying to say how they've made advances in chemo and radiation—I mean I don't know what advances, but I keep hearing about them. And she said no, that her body's too tired, that she's lived a good life and she doesn't want to go through that. And at that point, it was the weirdest feeling in me; it was almost like, you know, if all the windows were open in a house and all of a sudden, they all started closing and I couldn't catch my breath. I almost couldn't think anymore, there was so little air. And I just said, "If that's what you decide, then that's your right" and she said, "Thank you for respecting that" and we hung up.

THERAPIST 43: I would imagine that was a difficult moment for you.

CLIENT 43: Yes, it was, and I was just looking, you know, at the phone in my hand like, that's it. Then I figured well, the next day or a week from then, I would be able to get it together, ummm, but we didn't talk for a week after that and like, you know, she's typically over at the house at least twice a week.

THERAPIST 44: A week, not talking at all. That seems like a long time for you, right?

CLIENT 44: Yeah, I've only got a few months with her probably.

THERAPIST 45: Yeah, that's a hard one to get your head around. I think with that kind of diagnosis, it sounds like she was very direct with you about what she wanted. I really liked the way you described feeling like the windows were closing, and in particular that was helpful when you described how it's like there wasn't any air. And then, tell me if I'm on track here, but it sounded to me like it wasn't just how you thought about her decision, it was a whole embodied experience, like there wasn't enough here to really breathe. (Skill 6: Reinforcement of Effective Communication, reinforce how this effective communication positively influences the client's ability to be understood by the therapist)

CLIENT 45: That's exactly it—something I felt in my body way more than having any kind of rational thought. That's for sure.

THERAPIST 46: Okay, if I were to ask you to describe some of your emotions, what words would you use? What emotional experience did you have in that moment at home when the air kind of got sucked out? (Skill 7: Communication Analysis, ask the client about the emotions they experienced during the interpersonal incident)

CLIENT 46: I was terrified. And it's almost like, you know, before I think I might have said, like I was angry or frustrated with her, but thinking back to it now, that's not what it was. I was terrified and pleading.

THERAPIST 47: Oh, I see you were terrified, and it felt like you were pleading with her.

CLIENT 47: Right, that's more what it was.

THERAPIST 48: Yeah, feeling terrified and pleading resonates with you.

CLIENT 48: "Please, please try to find a way to stick around longer!" was what I was trying to say, but, yeah, the way that probably came out for me was different . . .

THERAPIST 49: How do you think it came out in the conversation?

CLIENT 49: I think it was more like frustrated or angry or something?

THERAPIST 50: Yeah, but it sounds like, if I'm understanding correctly, that in the moment, it was really a sense of just being terrified, and then overtime it kind of morphed into where it got expressed more as being frustrated or angry at her in some ways. (Skill 7: Communication Analysis, ask the client about the emotions they experienced during the interpersonal incident)

CLIENT 50: And then it's weird. Just when you think you're a grown up, you realize about a week later that I hadn't even thought about what it's like to have the diagnosis from her experience. I only thought about myself for a whole week. Like a child.

THERAPIST 51: That's a powerful recognition, to be able to see a situation from another person's perspective.

CLIENT 51: I mean, my sister had called me about 4 or 5 days after that first phone call to tell me to get my act together. And she was right. And then I kind of snapped to it and realized what it must be like from mom's point of view?

THERAPIST 52: Yeah. Again, very helpful. What were you hoping would have happened in that conversation? (Skill 7: Communication Analysis, ask the client what they were expecting and hoping to get from the other person in the specific incident)

CLIENT 52: The first one where she told me or the one a week later?

THERAPIST 53: The first one.

CLIENT 53: The first one . . . what I was hoping was that she'd realized how much we'll miss her. Umm, that by saying, you know, don't skip treatment that she'd realize we all want her to be around. I guess that's what I was hoping for. And so if she could have seen my intentions, I guess that's what I was hoping she would have understood.

THERAPIST 54: I see. So, based on what you're describing and literally what you just said, it seems to me that you're able to communicate what it is you're wanting and what your feelings are. You actually did beautifully just now. But if you're able to communicate that to her, that might help change that response. It might help you to kind of find a middle ground or understand each other's perspectives. Does that make sense? (Skill 7: Communication Analysis, suggest that an improved communication may lead to different results)

CLIENT 54: So much, you know, I can't imagine how it would have gone differently if I had said I'm terrified that you might be gone soon.

THERAPIST 55: If you would have said what you were actually thinking and feeling in that moment?

CLIENT 55: Right. You know how you always wish in the moment you would say something smart. If instead of being angry, I had said that I'm terrified of what it might be like without you and I can't imagine how you're feeling. I mean, right?

THERAPIST 56: Right, if you would have communicated your thoughts and feelings behind anger.

CLIENT 56: That was a million miles from my thoughts, and I didn't even think of getting to that second part until my sister called me 5 days later and told me to get my act together and get outside of my own head.

THERAPIST 57: Yeah. So one of the things that I'm curious about is if you had it to do over again—and you've kind of alluded to this—but if you had it to do over again, what would you have done differently? (Skill 7: Communication Analysis, suggest that improved communication may lead to different results)

CLIENT 57: I would have just stayed quiet for maybe a second or two. Umm. And, instead of just blurting out something. Now that I think about it, it was weird what came out of my mouth. Uh, what came out sounded angry.

THERAPIST 58: And you were feeling terrified.

CLIENT 58: Oh . . . like I was blocking it, you know.

THERAPIST 59: And instead the anger and frustration came out . . .

CLIENT 59: That's definitely right. What a thing to say in that moment. If I had a chance to do it over, I would take a breath and say, "It's going to take a little bit for me to figure out how I'm feeling, and it might even take me longer to be helpful to you, but I'm gonna try."

THERAPIST 60: Yeah, that sounds much closer to what you want to communicate, you know, and you gotta say, in a moment like that, especially when you're caught off guard completely by news like that, it's pretty tough to take that deep breath, especially, as you described, the air gets sucked out of the room and you just respond. (Skill 8: Generating Communication Options, provide feedback to the client about their proposed communication option)

CLIENT 60: Yeah, there was no breath to be had.

THERAPIST 61: So I think your response is very understandable, but clearly not really getting to the depth of what you wanted to share with her. What do you imagine might happen if you were to say something to your mom like, "You know, I really wish I would have said some additional things when we first had that conversation and you shared with me that you had cancer," how do you think she might respond to that? (Skill 8: Generating Communication Options, provide feedback to the client about their proposed communication option)

CLIENT 61: Almost like going back to her for a do over, huh? Uh. She would probably be surprised and relieved and grateful.

THERAPIST 62: Hmm. What do you imagine she might say specifically?

CLIENT 62: Like for real?

THERAPIST 63: Yeah.

CLIENT 63: What she might say . . . she might say, I love you. I've been so worried about you.

THERAPIST 64: Wow, that's—given the situation she's in, what an amazing thing for her to be able to say.

CLIENT 64: Yeah.

THERAPIST 65: Borrowing your words, if she heard "So I really want to do that over again because I felt like I came across as being really harsh, and gosh, it felt to me like, well, there wasn't any air to breathe. And so what I'd really like to say is that I'm scared and I'm really wanting to be supportive. I want to know what your experience is too, so I can understand that better." How do you think she'd respond to that? (Skill 8 Generating Communication Options, practice the proposed communication option using role-playing)

CLIENT 65: You know, she's always kind of worried about me. In a weird way, I think it would make her less worried about me. In a weird way, I think she would feel proud.

THERAPIST 66: Yeah. Would you mind if we actually did some role-playing in session? Maybe to practice just a bit.

CLIENT 66: I think anything that would make it so that I don't have to think on the spot would be good. If practicing helps, then I'm in.

THERAPIST 67: Usually when I do role-playing, I like to give some suggestions on how to communicate things first. Would that be okay if I imagine being you and you can imagine how your mom might respond?

CLIENT 67: That would be great.

THERAPIST 68: I might say this again: "So, uh, you know, Mom, I—I feel like I'd really like to have a do-over of the first conversation we had when you told me you had a cancer diagnosis." (Skill 8: Generating Communication Options, practice the proposed communication option using role-playing)

CLIENT 68: "I'd like that too. I know that must have been hard for you. It sure was hard for me."

THERAPIST 69: "But that's one of the things I've come to understand too is I was pretty much inside my own head there and then just really scared when I got that news. And since then, I've had a chance to just try and imagine things. What it's like for you to be dealing with that diagnosis and your own death. Oh, and I feel like I really missed the chance, and I'm afraid that what I said came across as being pretty harsh and that's not at all how I intended it." (Skill 8: Generating Communication Options, practice the proposed communication option using role-playing)

CLIENT 69: She would probably say, "That warms my heart more than you can imagine. For me, every day now is a gift, and I'm gonna unwrap it and enjoy it. Uh, and you know that I love to sing and play with your kids; this is giving me as much joy as that."

THERAPIST 70: Yeah. Well, it sounds like from the way you describe your mom, all you need to do is just open that door, and she'll be really receptive and appreciative. But nonetheless, would you mind if we try it the other way around? So if I were you and I threw out a couple of ideas, how would you improve on what I was suggesting? (Skill 8: Generating Communication Options, practice the proposed communication option using role-playing)

CLIENT 70: No, I liked what I heard so much and it's weird, I liked it and I sort of forgot the details of it. So I'll try to remember it because it's still hard for me to actually say it. Here goes: "So, Mom, I wanted to see if we could have a do-over from that very first conversation when you let me know about your cancer? Uh . . . I wish I'd handled that differently."

THERAPIST 71: "I appreciate you saying that. I was really worried about you after that conversation, so yeah, thanks for saying something." (Skill 8: Generating Communication Options, practice the proposed communication option using role-playing)

CLIENT 71: "I hate to be a burden, especially at a time like this. It's just that, umm, I was terrified—no lie. Umm, but, I didn't even ask how you were doing. And that's a big thing. I wanna—I wanna also be able to be there to help you too. . . . But I'm still terrified."

THERAPIST 72: "Well, thanks for saying something. That's got to be scary for you. And for your brother and sister too. And your babies. Umm, I'm going to miss being here too. But I want you to know that I really care about all of you and love you all very, very much." (Skill 8: Generating Communication Options, practice the proposed communication option using role-playing)

CLIENT 72: Could you imagine? Could you imagine if the call went that well? Oh my God. But yeah, I'm starting to actually be able to imagine it, right?

THERAPIST 73: You know, sometimes there's not a whole lot more that needs to be said. Sometimes it's just fundamental to give each other a hug.

CLIENT 73: Right.

THERAPIST 74: Yeah, that was nicely done. I think the way you opened the door there will let that communication happen.

CLIENT 74: And even as we're saying it out loud, it might be a better conversation in person than over the phone.

THERAPIST 75: Umm, well, we can't give somebody a hug over the phone so, you might be on to something there to have this conversation in person.

CLIENT 75: I don't even know the emoji.

THERAPIST 76: Yeah, well, the emojis are not the same either. I would strongly encourage you to have that conversation in person. I think that would be much better and help you to align your intentions with the projected impact.

CLIENT 76: Got it.

THERAPIST 77: So, that looks like it would work but let's increase the odds. What kind of support do you need to have that conversation? You know, would it be helpful to talk to your brother ahead of time, for instance, if you're ready for it? Is there anybody else you'd like to be there or not when you're having that conversation and when you could imagine doing that? (Skill 9: Mobilizing Social Support, collaboratively clarify the client's interpersonal support needs)

CLIENT 77: You know, I was thinking all I need to be able to have that conversation is for 3 days in a row to occur with nothing at all going wrong.

THERAPIST 78: OK, let me rephrase that. What's realistically a good time?

CLIENT 78: Well, instead of waiting for fate to deal me 3 perfect days, maybe it is smart to figure out who to lean on ahead of time. And yeah, I think it is my brother. One of the kinds of inside jokes we used to have with each other when we were teenagers was he would say he's my corner man. If I was in an argument with someone, like a girlfriend, and things got heated, I would go back to him and talk about it and he would say he felt like a corner man in a boxing match.

THERAPIST 79: I see, so he would support you.

CLIENT 79: Yes, so he's my corner man. So yeah, I could talk to him.

THERAPIST 80: Excellent and would it be helpful actually to have him there, or would that take away from the intensity of the experience you want to have with your mom? (Skill 9: Mobilizing Social Support, direct the client to engage specific people in their social support network to meet their needs)

CLIENT 80: Oh wow. Yes and yes. It probably makes it more likely to go well if he's there, but it does take away that intensity. But it would, you know, having him there, it's probably gonna be the smarter bet. Because yeah, even as I'm thinking it would depend on 3 days with nothing going wrong. It would also depend on, you know, my mom. I know it sounds like I've described a saint, but she's got looks on her face that sometimes make me think that I'm tiring for her also and if I see that, then I will start to worry that I'm exhausting for her. Yeah, I think my brother being there is a good idea.

THERAPIST 81: Okay, sounds like it's a good plan to have him there.

CLIENT 81: Just in case I start to spiral.

THERAPIST 82: Yeah. Yeah, sounds like that's a great idea. Would you mind if I gave you a couple of direct suggestions then?

CLIENT 82: I'd love it.

THERAPIST 83: So I really like the corner man analogy. Especially because the way I'm thinking about it visually is it's like you go into the ring and the going gets tough, and you go back and your corner man sometimes actually pushes you back out for the next round. (Skill 10: Motivating Interpersonal Action, reflect and enhance the client's readiness to engage in a new interpersonal action)

CLIENT 83: Right.

THERAPIST 84: Umm, so I can imagine that it would be tempting if the conversation is not going well for you to do what you describe doing: pulling back and not addressing it directly. But it might be very helpful to give your corner man some suggestions or directions on what you want him to do. (Skill 10: Motivating Interpersonal Action, reflect and enhance the client's readiness to engage in a new interpersonal action)

CLIENT 84: Right.

THERAPIST 85: Like, I want you just to be there. Not saying anything, but if you sense me kind of pulling back, then maybe even literally, you know, give me a push to keep going. (Skill 10: Motivating Interpersonal Actions, encourage a specific interpersonal action the client can implement)

CLIENT 85: Yeah, because my tendency is to walk away. I mean it's the same way when we were first talking on the phone. It just ended up, you know, clicking out. I mean, not hanging up on her, but still kind of clicking out easily, but that's not too different than just walking away. And so yeah, he would keep me from looking away.

THERAPIST 86: Okay. So it sounds to me like you've got a pretty good plan in place. I like the way you were thinking about starting the conversation with your mom. Having your brother there in the background, but to kind of serve as a backup, I think it makes it much more likely that that's going to happen. And by the way, there will be other opportunities for you once you get going to have a conversation with her individually too. That sounds like a great plan. So when could you do that? (Skill 10: Motivating Interpersonal Action, reflect and enhance the client's readiness to engage in a new interpersonal action)

CLIENT 86: Oh. Well, my brother wants to plan vacation time with his family and her, like a long weekend. That's in 2 weeks, so it's got to be before then.

THERAPIST 87: Yes, sounds like having the conversation sooner would be more helpful.

CLIENT 87: Uh, because, yeah, we don't know what we don't know, like in terms of how much time we've got. What's today? I'll have to call him and see if he's got time. She's over a lot at one of our houses, so it could even be when she's at their house. No wait, not in front of his kids or mine. Well, my kids could be with, uh, their mom. That's an advantage at least to having two homes. I would think in the next few days.

THERAPIST 88: Okay. So if you were to give yourself a homework assignment between now and next time we meet, what would it be? (Skill 10: Motivating Interpersonal Action, reflect and enhance the client's readiness to engage in a new interpersonal action)

CLIENT 88: I mean, call my corner man and set this up, figure out whether it'll be in my house or his. Set it up so that we could have this conversation in a way that not everyone else is around. You know, maybe the more I'm saying it, maybe it's his house. Yeah, my homework is to arrange it even if it doesn't happen this week to set it up.

THERAPIST 89: Yeah, that sounds great. That's a wonderful first step. I would encourage you, if possible, to have that conversation too. I think you're set to go with that. It's gonna be hard to get it started, but I think once you open the door, your mom will respond well. I think getting it set up sounds great, and then later, if you can have that conversation with her too, that would be great. What do you think about that? (Skill 10: Motivating Interpersonal Action, reflect and enhance the client's readiness to engage in a new interpersonal action)

CLIENT 89: It'll be such a relief to be able to do this. It would be such a relief. It will give me peace of mind.

THERAPIST 90: Yes, it will.

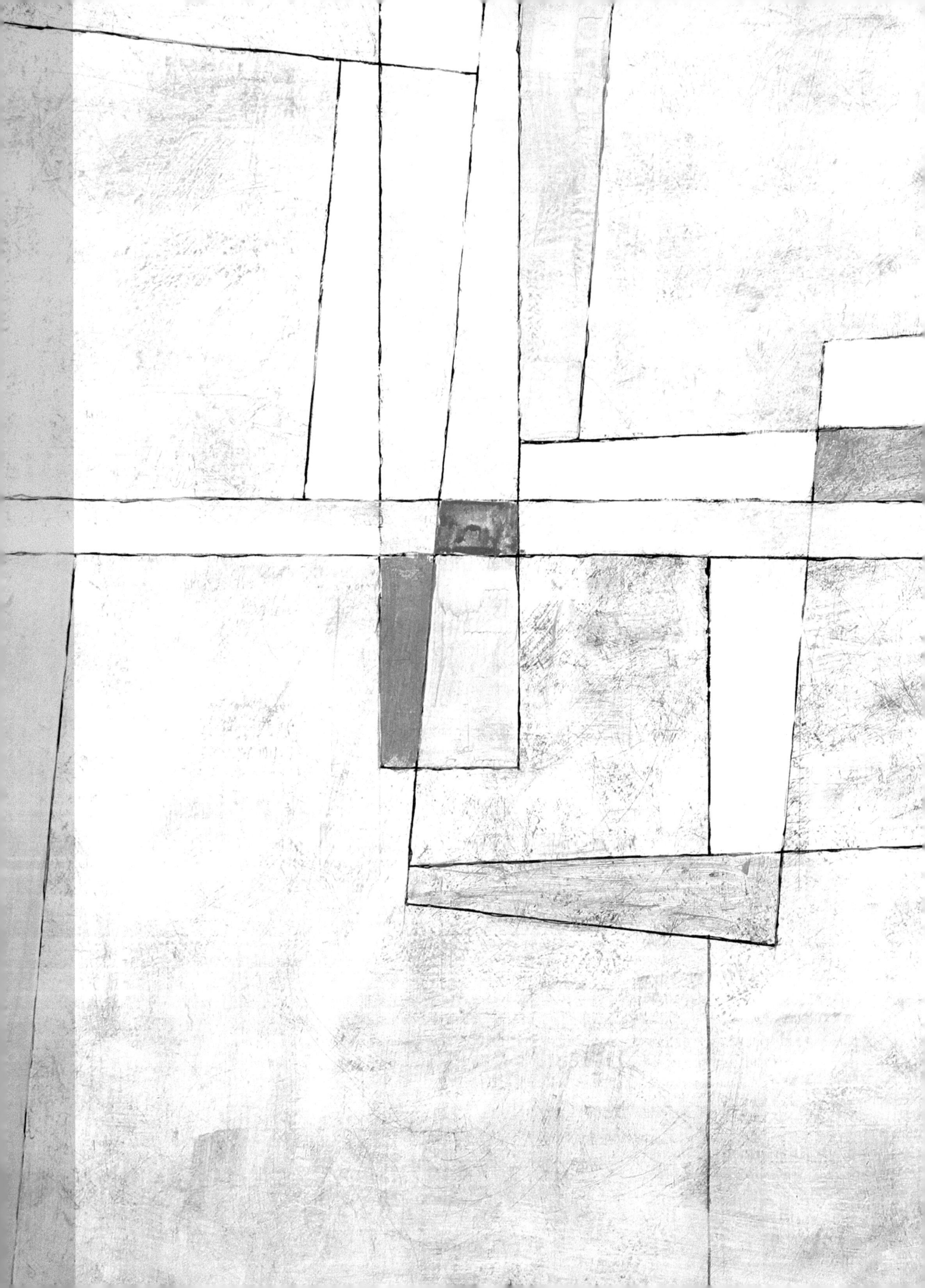

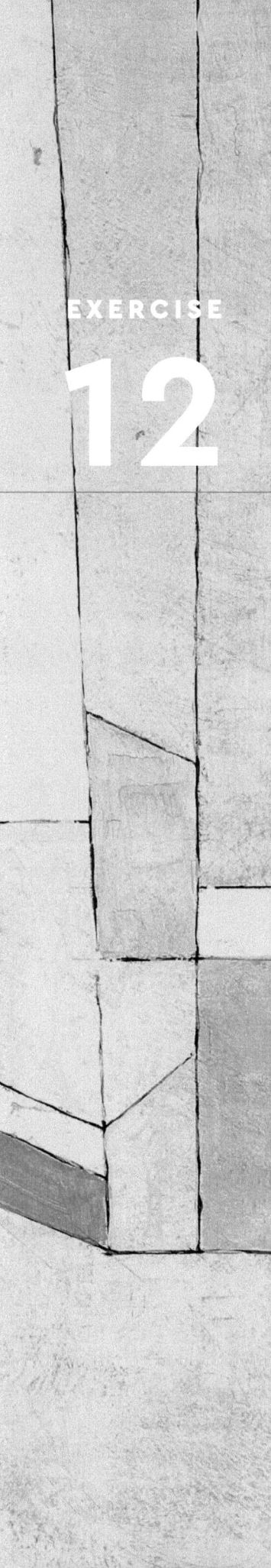

Mock Interpersonal Psychotherapy Sessions

In contrast to highly structured and repetitive deliberate practice exercises, a mock interpersonal psychotherapy (IPT) session is an unstructured and improvised role-play therapy session. Like a jazz rehearsal, mock sessions let you practice the art and science of *appropriate responsiveness* (Hatcher, 2015; Stiles & Horvath, 2017), putting your psychotherapy skills together in a way that is helpful to your mock client. This exercise outlines the procedure for conducting a mock IPT session. It offers different client profiles you may choose to adopt when role-playing the client.

Mock sessions are an opportunity for trainees to practice the following:

- using psychotherapy skills responsively
- navigating challenging choice-points in therapy
- choosing which interventions to use
- tracking the arc of a therapy session and the overall big-picture therapy treatment
- guiding treatment in the context of the client's preferences
- determining realistic goals for therapy in the context of the client's capacities
- knowing how to proceed when the therapist is unsure, lost, or confused
- recognizing and recovering from therapeutic errors
- discovering your personal therapeutic style
- building endurance for working with real clients

Mock Interpersonal Psychotherapy Session Overview

For the mock session, **you will perform a role-play of an initial therapy session**. As is true with the exercises to build individual skills, the role-play involves three people: One trainee role-plays the therapist, another trainee role-plays the client, and a trainer (a professor or a supervisor) observes and provides feedback. This is an open-ended role-play, as is commonly done in training. However, this differs in two important ways

https://doi.org/10.1037/0000426-014

Deliberate Practice in Interpersonal Psychotherapy, by O. Belik, J. M. Schultz, S. Fairhurst, S. Stuart, A. Vaz, and T. Rousmaniere

from the role-plays used in more traditional training. First, the therapist will use their hand to indicate how difficult the role-play feels. Second, the client will attempt to make the role-play easier or harder to ensure the therapist is practicing at the right difficulty level.

Preparation

1. Download the Deliberate Practice Reaction Form and the Deliberate Practice Diary Form from the "Resources" tab at https://www.apa.org/pubs/books/deliberate-practice-interpersonal-psychotherapy (also available in Appendixes A and B, respectively). Every student will need their own copy of the Deliberate Practice Reaction Form on a separate piece of paper so they can access it quickly.

2. Designate one student to role-play the therapist and one student to role-play the client. The trainer will observe and provide corrective feedback.

Mock Interpersonal Psychotherapy Session Procedure

1. The trainees will role-play an initial (first) therapy session. The trainee role-playing the client selects a client profile from the end of this exercise.

2. Before beginning the role-play, the therapist raises their hand to their side, at the level of their chair seat (see Figure E12.1). They will use this hand throughout the role-play to indicate how challenging it feels to them to help the client. Their starting hand level (chair seat) indicates that the role-play feels easy. By raising their hand, the therapist

FIGURE E12.1. Ongoing Difficulty Assessment Through Hand Level

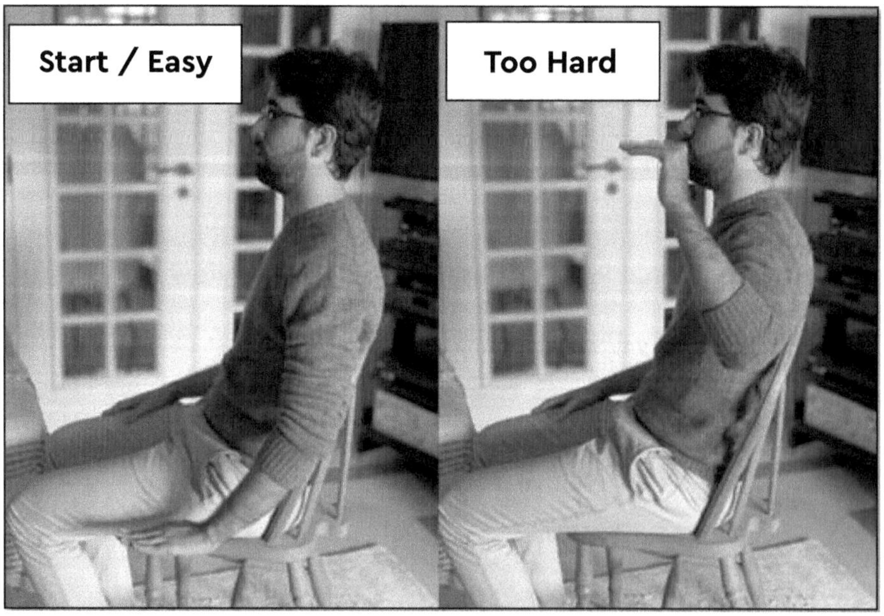

Note. Left: Start of role-play. Right: Role-play is too difficult. From *Deliberate Practice in Emotion-Focused Therapy* (p. 156), by R. N. Goldman, A. Vaz, and T. Rousmaniere, 2021, American Psychological Association (https://doi.org/10.1037/0000227-000). Copyright 2021 by the American Psychological Association.

indicates that the difficulty is rising. If their hand rises above their neck level, it indicates that the role-play is too difficult.

3. The therapist begins the role-play. The therapist and client should engage in the role-play in an improvised manner, as they would engage in a real therapy session. The therapist keeps their hand out at their side throughout this process. (This may feel strange at first!)

4. Whenever the therapist feels that the difficulty of the role-play has changed significantly, they should move their hand up if it feels more difficult, down if it feels easier. If the therapist's hand drops below the seat of their chair, the client should make the role-play more challenging; if the therapist's hand rises above their neck level, the client should make the role-play easier. Instructions for adjusting the difficulty of the role-play are described in the Varying the Level of Challenge section later in the exercise.

Note to Therapists

Remember to be aware of your vocal quality. Match your tone to the client's presentation. Thus, if the client presents vulnerable, soft emotions behind their words, soften your tone to be soothing and calm. If, on the other hand, the client is aggressive and angry, match your tone to be firm and solid. If you choose responses that are prompting of client exploration, such as the Interpersonal Inventory (Exercise 2), remember to adopt a more querying, exploratory tone of voice.

5. The role-play continues for at least 15 minutes. The trainer may provide corrective feedback during this process if the therapist gets significantly off track. However, trainers should exercise restraint and keep feedback as short and tight as possible because too much feedback will reduce the therapist's opportunity for experiential training.

6. After the role-play is finished, the therapist and client switch roles and begin a new mock session.

7. After both trainees have completed the mock session as a therapist, the trainees and the trainer discuss the experience.

Varying the Level of Challenge

If the therapist indicates that the mock session is too easy, the person enacting the role of the client can use the following modifications to make it more challenging (see also Appendix A):

- The client can improvise with topics that are more evocative or make the therapist uncomfortable, such as expressing currently held strong feelings (see Figure A.2).
- The client can use a distressed voice (e.g., angry, sad, sarcastic) or unpleasant facial expression. This increases the emotional tone.
- Blend complex mixtures of opposing feelings (e.g., love and rage).
- Become confrontational, questioning the purpose of therapy or the therapist's fitness for the role.

If the therapist indicates that the mock session is too hard:

- The client can be guided by Figure A.2 to
  - present topics that are less evocative,
  - present material on any topic but without expressing feelings, or
  - present material concerning the future or the past or events outside therapy.
- The client can ask the questions in a soft voice or with a smile. This softens the emotional stimulus.
- The therapist can take short breaks during the role-play.
- The trainer can expand the "feedback phase" by discussing IPT or psychotherapy theory.

Mock Session Client Profiles

Following are six client profiles for trainees to use during mock sessions, presented in order of difficulty. The choice of client profile may be determined by the trainee playing the therapist, determined by the trainee playing the client, or assigned by the trainer.

The most important aspect of role-plays is for trainees to convey the emotional tone indicated by the client profile (e.g., "angry," "sad"). The demographics of the client (e.g., age, gender) and specific content of the client profiles are not important. Thus, trainees should adjust the client profile to be most comfortable and easy for the trainee to role-play. For example, a trainee may change the client profile from female to male, from 45 to 22 years old, and so on.

Beginner Profile: Communication Skills and Grief and Loss

Marianna is a 47-year-old Latina lesbian cisgender female whose mother was diagnosed with cancer 3 months ago. Marianna's mother just informed her family that she will not be seeking medical treatment and asked all the family members to respect her decision. There have been no additional conversations between Marianna and her mother about her medical diagnosis since her mother made an announcement 3 months ago. Marianna has been experiencing sadness and anxiety about the upcoming loss of her mother. In addition, she has been feeling angry about her mother's decision and indicated that she feels "confused and shocked" by the decision. Marianna is married and has two teenage children with her wife of 20 years. She describes her marriage and her wife as "very loving, supporting, and understanding." Marianna came to treatment asking for help processing her sadness, upcoming loss, and anger about her mother's decision to not seek medical treatment. She is also asking for guidance about communicating with her mother as she is reporting "not knowing" how to initiate the conversation about her mother's health and wanting to say "many things" but not knowing exactly "what to say or how to say it."

- **Symptoms:** Sadness, confusion, and anger

- **Client's goals for therapy:** Marianna wants to process her complex feelings about her mother's diagnosis and decision to not seek medical treatment as well as assistance with initiating and constructing a conversation and communication with her mother.

- **Attitude toward therapy:** Marianna has never been in therapy before and comes in highly motivated and open to explore and understand her feelings and intentions, as well as to learn new communication skills.

- **Strengths:** Marianna is very motivated to engage in therapeutic work, has strong and stable interpersonal support, and is open with the therapist.

Beginner Profile: Role Transitions

Henry is a 23-year-old Black, cisgender male graduate student who moved to a big city after being accepted into law school at a prestigious university. This has been a huge transition for Henry because he had to move away from his family and friends and start law school. Henry lived in the same city all his life, knows and feels "being known" by a lot of people there. He has never been away from his support for a prolonged period of time. He loves his program and is doing well academically, but he feels lonely and a bit "lost" in the big city without the support system that he is used to. He is reporting sadness as he is missing his family and friends more than he initially thought he would. He is finding it challenging to find friends as most of his classmates, including himself, are busy with academic studies. He is coming to therapy because he noticed feeling sad and lonely and is starting to question his decision to move away from his support system. He is interested in continuing his graduate studies and learning ways to make new friends.

- **Symptoms:** Feeling lonely and sad and experiencing lack of social support

- **Client's goals for therapy:** Henry is coming in asking for assistance in understanding his feelings and obtaining new skills in initiating new relationships. He is highly motivated to make meaningful connections with other people that can turn into mutually supportive friendships.

- **Attitude toward therapy:** Henry has never been in therapy before but knows some friends "back home" who found therapy "helpful." He is hopeful that this will help him as well.

- **Strengths:** Henry is engaged and motivated to participate in the therapeutic work.

Intermediate Profile: Interpersonal Disputes With Friends

Isabella is a 15-year-old White cisgender female who is having a difficult time "fitting in" with her friends at school. She is doing well academically and is on a school's sports team. She indicates that lately it has been challenging to maintain some friendships because "all they do is gossip about other people." She is feeling sad that she no longer has close relationships with some of her "friends" and recently left a group chat "because they started saying mean things about some of the teachers and other students at school." This decision triggered a dispute between her and her friends that she is still trying to resolve. Isabella has an older sister who has been a source of support and guidance to her. Isabella was referred to therapy by her mother, who noticed Isabella's sad mood in the past month or so. Isabella agreed to participate in therapy and stated that it would help her "to understand the situation and her friends better." She is also looking for communication skills that would potentially help her initiate new relationships.

- **Symptoms:** Sadness, social withdrawal, and loneliness

- **Client's goals for therapy:** Isabella wants to make sense of the current interpersonal disputes with her "friends" and potentially gain skills to initiate new friendships.

- **Attitude toward therapy:** Although Isabella did not self-refer to therapy, she indicated that it will be helpful to her given what is "going on at school with her friends."

- **Strengths:** Isabella appears to be confident in knowing her relational values and aspects of friendship that she prefers to see with others.

Intermediate Profile: Role Transitions Related to the Loss of Health

Jeff is a 20-year-old Asian American cisgender male who was referred to therapy by his primary care physician. Jeff was recently diagnosed with a medical condition that would preclude him from playing basketball with his friends on a weekly basis. He has been playing basketball with his group of friends and coworkers for the past 5 years every weekend, and their friendships have been getting stronger. Jeff is worried that he will sustain the loss of his relationships with his basketball team. He does not have a lot of friends or support outside of his basketball team. He is worried about his diagnosis and everyday adjustments, including medical treatment, that he will have to make.

- **Symptoms:** Anxiety; sadness; and worries about relationships, health, and general lifestyle

- **Client's goals for therapy:** Jeff wants to address the changes that he is starting to go through. He wants to understand his emotions and learn how to communicate the transitions to other people in his life.

- **Attitude toward therapy:** Jeff had been in therapy for anxiety treatment when he was a teenager. He hopes that therapy will help him again this time.

- **Strengths:** Jeff is engaged and committed to therapeutic process and work.

Advanced Profile: Role Transitions and Interpersonal Dispute

Audre is a 39-year-old Black bisexual female veteran who recently returned to civilian life. She is recently divorced and currently going through infertility treatment with her female partner. She sustained sexual trauma while she was in the military. She is presenting with trauma symptoms, anxiety about transition to civilian life, employment, and her health as it relates to her ability to become pregnant. She reports a good relationship with her partner, whom she describes as "supportive and understanding," but is currently having difficult time with her family members, especially her mother, who is not fully supportive of Audre having a child with her partner. Disputes with her mother are affecting her relationship with her partner and "stressing her out" in general. In addition, all three of her adult siblings tend to go to her for any help they might need, and Audre is "starting to feel overwhelmed."

- **Symptoms:** Trauma symptoms, anxiety, interpersonal disputes with family, adjustment to civilian life, and health concerns

- **Client's goals for therapy:** Audre is interested in addressing trauma and anxiety symptoms and the impact they have on her interpersonal functioning. She is also interested in addressing her current transition to civilian life and becoming a mother. Audre wishes to resolve family-related interpersonal disputes.

- **Attitude toward therapy:** Audre attended therapy when she was in elementary school and does not recall it being helpful. She is ambivalent about the therapeutic process and indicated that she has "trust issues" toward any authority. During the intake, she stated that she is "willing to give therapy a try."

- **Strengths:** Audre is dedicated to improving her mental health. She is extremely resilient and has strong support from her partner. She loves her family and is invested in the resolution of interpersonal dispute.

Advanced Profile: Family Transitions and Interpersonal Disputes With Peers

Alex is a 13-year-old White male who is experiencing bullying at school and was referred to therapy by a school counselor. His parents are in the process of separation, and he recently started to live in two households, changing his residency between parents weekly. He was in therapy when he was 7 years old for depression, anxiety, and witnessing domestic violence at home. He was temporarily removed from his home at that time and was reunited with his parents after being in foster care for 4 months. While in foster care, he was emotionally abused by another foster child. He is currently reporting sadness, worrying, and difficulties falling and sustaining sleep. He is "afraid" about the possibility of going back to foster care. He minimizes the bullying, saying, "it's okay" and states that he does not know how to stand up for himself. When he does speak up for himself, it leads to verbal or physical fights with his peers. He has some friends at school but does not see them outside of the school. He is close to his maternal grandmother who lives not far from his parents.

- **Symptoms:** Sadness, anxiety, bullying, and changes and transitions within the family structure

- **Client's goals for therapy:** Alex wants to have more friends and for the bullying to stop. He wants his parents to be together and indicated that "maybe if he makes some changes," his parents might get back together.

- **Attitude toward therapy:** Alex was in therapy before and is willing to participate again.

- **Strengths:** Alex has a good awareness of his feelings and can narrate his feelings and thoughts when assisted and asked.

Advanced Interpersonal Psychotherapy Profile: Play Yourself

The last profile suggests that therapists in training play themselves and choose a relational situation that brought about distress of an interpersonal nature for them. It is important for the person playing client to choose a personal issue or topic that they feel comfortable discussing and further exploring. We recommend they monitor their own experience during this training opportunity and thoughtfully choose what and how much they wish to disclose.

This in vivo training approach provides an opportunity for the trainee to practice and further sharpen their ability to perceive their actual experience. Through the engagement in metacognitions, the trainee can actively calibrate, in the moment, their working clinical hypothesis. As they test their clinical rationale and approaches with immediate feedback, they get an opportunity to feel the impact of the various responses and evaluate, from moment to moment, the impact of IPT.

Lastly, part of the competency in IPT is clinicians' own interpersonal skills and ability to navigate clinically complicated situations, which requires awareness of our own perceptions, needs, and emotional preferences. When you choose to draw on your actual experience as a client, you learn an immense amount about what might or might not be helpful to you. Understanding your preferences can help you further differentiate your own needs from those of a client, which in return can assist in obtaining an objective clinical stance in IPT.

Instructions

Work in pairs. One trainee playing the client chooses an issue from their own life that they wish to discuss and feels comfortable to explore in the training setting.

Trainees may choose an issue that they have been struggling with recently and about which they want to obtain further clarification, problem solve, or gain specific communication skills that would assist with the chosen interpersonal situation. If you are playing yourself as a client, you may want to think over in advance (a) what relational problems or issues, symptoms, or behaviors you wish to discuss; (b) what your goal of the session might be (clarification could be a goal); and (c) what attitude toward your therapist you wish to convey (curiosity about your own experience is one option).

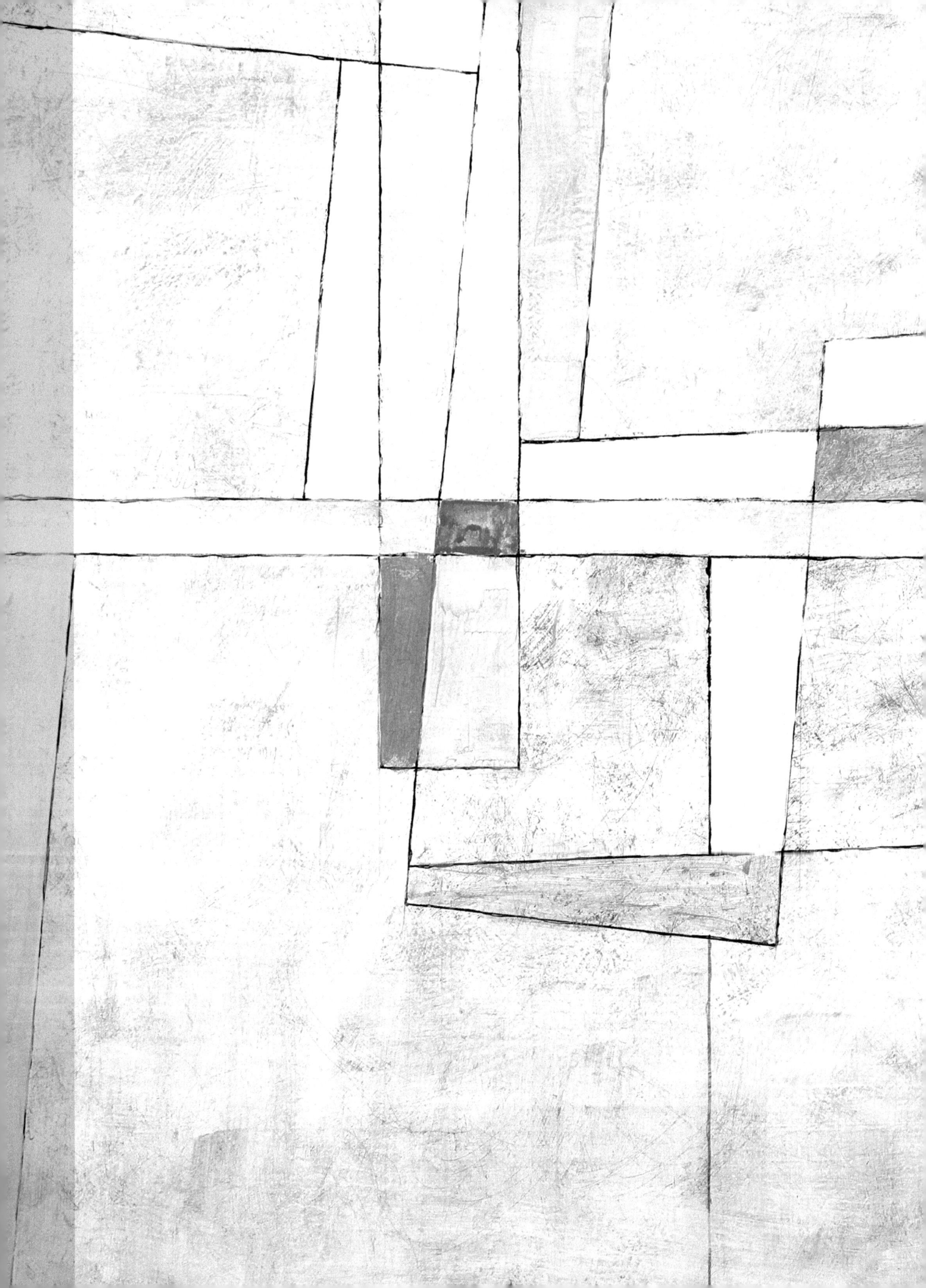

Strategies for Enhancing the Deliberate Practice Exercises

Part III consists of one chapter, Chapter 3, that provides additional advice and instructions for trainers and trainees so that they can reap more benefits from the deliberate practice exercises in Part II. Chapter 3 offers six key points for getting the most out of deliberate practice, guidelines for practicing appropriately responsive treatment, evaluation strategies, methods for ensuring trainee well-being and respecting their privacy, and advice for monitoring the trainer–trainee relationship.

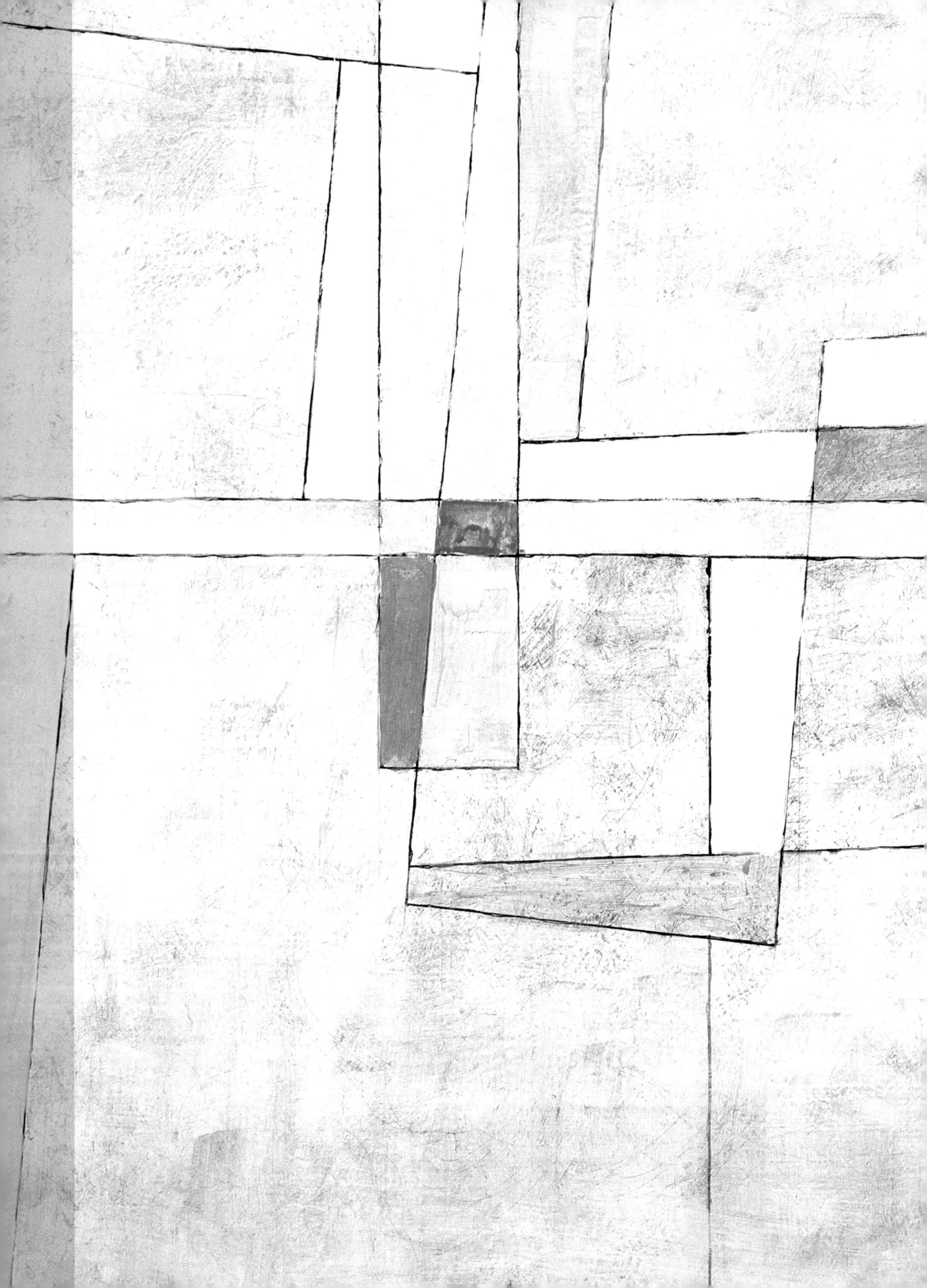

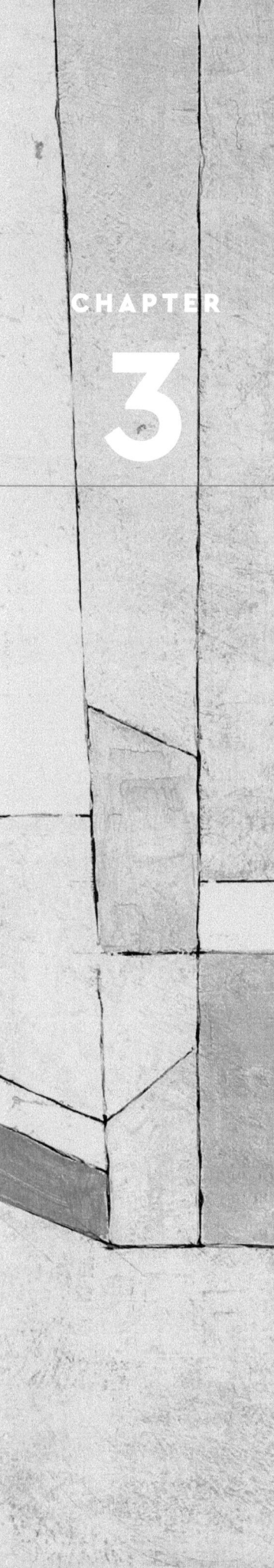

How to Get the Most Out of Deliberate Practice: Additional Guidance for Trainers and Trainees

In Chapter 2 and in the exercises themselves, we have provided instructions for completing the deliberate practice exercises. This chapter provides guidance on big-picture topics that trainers will need to integrate deliberate practice successfully into their training program. This guidance is based on relevant research and the experiences and feedback from trainers at more than a dozen psychotherapy training programs who volunteered to test the deliberate practice exercises in this book. We cover topics including evaluation, getting the most from deliberate practice, trainee well-being, respecting trainee privacy, trainer self-evaluation, responsive treatment, and the trainee–trainer alliance.

Six Key Points for Getting the Most From Deliberate Practice

Following are six key points of advice for trainers and trainees to get the most benefit from the interpersonal psychotherapy (IPT) deliberate practice exercises. The following advice is gleaned from experiences vetting and practicing the exercises, sometimes in different languages, with many trainees, across many countries.

Key Point 1: Create Realistic Emotional Stimuli

A key component of deliberate practice is using stimuli that provoke similar reactions to challenging real-life work settings. For example, pilots train with flight simulators that present mechanical failures and dangerous weather conditions; surgeons practice with surgical simulators that present medical complications with only seconds to respond. Training with challenging stimuli will increase trainees' capacity to perform therapy effectively under stress, for example with clients they find challenging. The stimuli used for IPT deliberate practice exercises are role-plays of challenging client statements in therapy. **It is important that the trainee who is role-playing the client performs the script with appropriate emotional expression and maintains eye contact with the therapist.** For example, if the client statement calls for sad emotion, the trainee

https://doi.org/10.1037/0000426-015

Deliberate Practice in Interpersonal Psychotherapy, by O. Belik, J. M. Schultz, S. Fairhurst, S. Stuart, A. Vaz, and T. Rousmaniere

should try to express sadness eye-to-eye with the therapist. We offer the suggestions regarding emotional expressiveness:

1. The emotional tone of the role-play matters more than the exact words of each script. Trainees role-playing the client should feel free to improvise and change the words if it will help them be more emotionally expressive. Trainees do not need to stick 100% exactly to the script. In fact, to read off the script during the exercise can sound flat and prohibit eye contact. Rather, trainees in the client role should first read the client statement silently to themselves, then, when ready, say it in an emotional manner while looking directly at the trainee playing the therapist. This will help the experience feel more real and engaging for the therapist.

2. Trainees whose first language isn't English may particularly benefit from reviewing and changing the words in the client statement script before each role-play so that they can find words that feel congruent and facilitate emotional expression.

3. Trainees role-playing the client should try to use tonal and nonverbal expressions of feelings. For example, if a script calls for anger, the trainee can speak with an angry voice and make fists with their hands; if a script calls for shame or guilt, the trainee could hunch over and wince; if a script calls for sadness, the trainee could speak in a soft or deflated voice.

4. If trainees are having persistent difficulties acting believably when following a particular script in the role of client, it may help to first do a "demo round" by reading directly from paper, and then, immediately after, dropping the paper to make eye contact and repeating the same client statement from memory. Some trainees reported this helped them "become available as real clients" and made the role-play feel less artificial. Some trainees did three or four "demo rounds" to get fully into their role as a client.

Key Point 2: Customize the Exercises to Fit Your Unique Training Circumstances

Deliberate practice is less about adhering to specific rules than it is about using training principles. Every trainer has their own individual teaching style and every trainee their own learning process. Thus, the exercises in this book are designed to be flexibly customized by trainers across different training contexts within different cultures. Trainees and trainers are encouraged to adjust exercises continually to optimize their practice. The most effective training will occur when deliberate practice exercises are customized to fit the learning needs of each trainee and culture of each training site. In our experience with numerous trainers and trainees across many countries, we found that everyone spontaneously customized the exercises for their unique training circumstances. No two trainers followed the exact same procedure. For example:

*   One supervisor used the exercises with a trainee who found all the client statements to be too hard, including the "beginner" stimuli. This trainee had multiple reactions in the "too hard" category, including nausea, severe shame, and self-doubt. The trainee disclosed to the supervisor that she had experienced extremely harsh learning environments earlier in her life and found the role-plays to be highly evocative. To help, the supervisor followed the suggestions offered in Appendix A to make the stimuli progressively easier until the trainee reported feeling "good challenge" on the Deliberate Practice Reaction Form. Over many weeks of practice, the trainee developed a sense of safety and was able to practice with more difficult client statements. (Note that if the supervisor had proceeded at the too hard difficulty level, the

trainee might have complied while hiding her negative reactions, become emotionally flooded and overwhelmed, leading to withdrawal and thus prohibiting her skill
development and risking dropout from training.)

- Supervisors of trainees for whom English was not their first language adjusted the
client statements to their own primary language.

- One supervisor used the exercises with a trainee who found all the stimuli to be
too easy, including the advanced client statements. This supervisor quickly moved
to improvising more challenging client statements from scratch by following the
instructions in Appendix A on how to make client statements more challenging.

Key Point 3: Discover Your Own Unique Personal Therapeutic Style

Deliberate practice in psychotherapy can be likened to the process of learning to play
jazz music. Every jazz musician prides themselves in their skillful improvisations, and
the process of "finding your own voice" is a prerequisite for expertise in jazz musi-
cianship. Yet improvisations are not a collection of random notes but the culmination
of extensive deliberate practice over time. Indeed, the ability to improvise is built on
many hours of dedicated practice of scales, melodies, harmonies, and so on. Much
in the same way, psychotherapy trainees are encouraged to experience the scripted
interventions in this book not as ends in themselves but as a means to promote skill in a
systematic fashion. Over time, effective therapeutic creativity can be aided, instead of
constrained, by dedicated practice in these therapeutic "melodies."

Key Point 4: Engage in a Sufficient Amount of Rehearsal

Deliberate practice uses rehearsal to move skills into procedural memory, which helps
trainees maintain access to skills even when working with challenging clients. This only
works if trainees engage in many repetitions of the exercises. Think of a challenging sport
or musical instrument you learned: How many rehearsals would a professional need to
feel confident performing a new skill? Psychotherapy is no easier than those other fields!

Key Point 5: Continually Adjust Difficulty

A crucial element of deliberate practice is training at an optimal difficulty level: neither
too easy nor too hard. To achieve this, do difficulty assessments and adjustments with
the Deliberate Practice Reaction Form in Appendix A. **Do not skip this step!** If trainees
don't feel any of the "good challenge" reactions at the bottom of the Deliberate Practice Reaction Form, then the exercise is probably too easy; if they feel any of the "too
hard" reactions then the exercise could be too difficult for the trainee to benefit.
Advanced trainees and therapists may find all the client statements too easy. If so, they
should follow the instructions in Appendix A on making client statements harder to
make the role-plays sufficiently challenging.

Key Point 6: Putting It All Together With the Practice Transcript and Mock Therapy Sessions

Some trainees may seek greater contextualization of the individual therapy responses
associated with each skill, feeling the need to integrate the disparate pieces of their
training in a more coherent manner with a simulation that mimics a real therapy session.
The annotated transcript in Exercise 11 and the mock therapy sessions in Exercise 12

give trainees this opportunity, allowing them to practice delivering different responses sequentially in a more realistic therapeutic encounter.

Responsive Treatment

The exercises in this book are designed not only to help trainees acquire specific skills of IPT, but to use them in ways that are responsive to each individual client. Across the psychotherapy literature, this stance has been referred to as *appropriate responsiveness*, wherein the therapists exercise flexible judgment, based in their perception of the client's emotional state, needs, and goals, and integrates techniques and other interpersonal skills in pursuit of optimal client outcomes (Hatcher, 2015; Stiles et al., 1998). The effective therapist is responsive to the emerging context. As Stiles and Horvath (2017) argued, therapists are effective because they are appropriately responsive. Doing the "right thing" may be different each time and means providing each client with an individually tailored response.

Appropriate responsiveness counters a misconception that deliberate practice rehearsal is designed to promote robotic repetition of therapy techniques. Psychotherapy researchers have shown that overadherence to a particular model while neglecting client preferences reduces therapy effectiveness (e.g., Castonguay et al., 1996; Henry et al., 1993; Owen & Hilsenroth, 2014). Therapist flexibility, on the other hand, has been shown to improve outcomes (e.g., Bugatti & Boswell, 2016; Kendall & Beidas, 2007; Kendall & Frank, 2018). It is important, therefore, that trainees practice their newly learned skills in a manner that is flexible and responsive to the unique needs of a diverse range of clients (Hatcher, 2015; Hill & Knox, 2013). It is thus of paramount importance for trainees to develop the necessary perceptual skills to be able to attune to what the client is experiencing in the moment and form their response based on the client moment-by-moment context (Greenberg & Goldman, 1988).

The supervisor must help the supervisee to specifically attune themselves to the unique and specific interpersonal needs of the clients during sessions. By enacting responsiveness with the supervisee, the supervisor can demonstrate its value and make it more explicit. In these ways, attention can be given to the larger picture of appropriate responsiveness. Here the trainee and supervisor can work together to help the trainee master not just the techniques but how therapists can use their judgment to put the techniques together to foster positive change. Helping trainees keep this overarching goal in mind while reviewing the therapy process is a valuable feature of supervision that is difficult to obtain otherwise (Hatcher, 2015).

It is also important that deliberate practice occurs within a context of wider IPT learning. As noted in Chapter 1, training should be combined with supervision of actual therapy recordings, theoretical learning, observation of competent IPT psychotherapists, as well as personal therapeutic work. When the trainer or trainee determines that the trainee is having difficulty acquiring IPT skills, it is important to assess carefully what is missing or needed. Assessment should then lead to the appropriate remedy, as the trainer and trainee collaboratively determine what is needed.

Being Mindful of Trainee Well-Being

Although negative effects that some clients experience in psychotherapy have been well documented (Barlow, 2010), negative effects of training and supervision on trainees have received less attention (Ellis et al., 2014). To support strong self-efficacy, trainers must ensure that trainees are practicing at a correct difficulty level. The exercises in this book feature guidance for frequently assessing and adjusting the difficulty level so that trainees can rehearse at a level that precisely targets their personal skill threshold. Trainers and supervisors must be mindful to provide an appropriate challenge. One risk to trainees that is particularly pertinent to this book occurs when using role-plays that are too difficult. The Deliberate Practice Reaction Form in Appendix A is provided to help trainers ensure that role-plays are done at an appropriate challenge level. Trainers or trainees may be tempted to skip the difficulty assessments and adjustments out of their motivation to focus on rehearsal to make fast progress and quickly acquire skills. But across all our test sites, we found that skipping the difficulty assessments and adjustments caused more problems and hindered skill acquisition more than any other error. Thus, trainers are advised to remember that **one of their most important responsibilities is to remind trainees to do the difficulty assessments and adjustments.**

Additionally, the Deliberate Practice Reaction Form serves a dual purpose of helping trainees develop the important skills of self-monitoring and self-awareness (Bennett-Levy, 2019). This will help trainees adopt a positive and empowered stance regarding their own self-care and should facilitate career-long professional development.

Respecting Trainee Privacy

The deliberate practice exercises in this book may stir up complex or uncomfortable personal reactions within trainees, including for example memories of past traumas. Exploring psychological and emotional reactions may make some trainees feel vulnerable. Therapists of every career stage, from trainees to seasoned therapists with decades of experience, commonly experience shame, embarrassment, and self-doubt in this process. Although these experiences can be valuable for building trainees' self-awareness, it is important that training remains focused on professional skill development and not blur into personal therapy (e.g., Ellis et al., 2014). Therefore, one trainer role is to remind trainees to maintain appropriate boundaries.

Trainees must have the final say about what to disclose or not disclose to their trainer. Trainees should keep in mind that the goal is for the trainee to expand their own self-awareness and psychological capacity to stay active and helpful while experiencing uncomfortable reactions. The trainer does not need to know the specific details about the trainee's inner world for this to happen.

Trainees should be instructed to disclose only personal information that they feel comfortable sharing. The Deliberate Practice Reaction Form and difficulty assessment process is designed to help trainees build their self-awareness while retaining control over their privacy. Trainees can be reminded that the goal is for them to learn about their own inner world. They do not necessarily have to share that information with trainers or peers (Bennett-Levy & Finlay-Jones, 2018). Likewise, trainees should be instructed to respect the confidentiality of their peers.

Trainer Self-Evaluation

The exercises in this book were tested at a wide range of training sites around the world, including graduate courses, practicum sites, and private practice offices. Although trainers reported that the exercises were highly effective for training, some also said that they felt disoriented by how different deliberate practice feels compared with their traditional methods of clinical education. Many felt comfortable evaluating their trainees' performance but were less sure about their own performance as trainers.

The most common concern we heard from trainers was, "My trainees are doing great, but I'm not sure if I am doing this correctly!" To address this concern, we recommend trainers perform periodic self-evaluations along the following five criteria:

1. Observe trainees' work performance.
2. Provide continual corrective feedback.
3. Ensure rehearsal of specific skills is just beyond the trainees' current ability.
4. Ensure that the trainee is practicing at the right difficulty level (neither too easy nor too challenging).
5. Continuously assess trainee performance with real clients.

Criterion 1: Observe Trainees' Work Performance

Determining how well we are doing as trainers means first having valid information about how well trainees are responding to training. This requires that we directly observe trainees practicing skills to provide corrective feedback and evaluation. One risk of deliberate practice is that trainees gain competence in performing therapy skills in role-plays, but those skills do not transfer to trainees' work with real clients. Thus, trainers will ideally also have the opportunity to observe samples of trainees' work with real clients, either live or via recorded video. Supervisors and consultants rely heavily—and, too often, exclusively—on supervisees' and consultees' narrative accounts of their work with clients (Goodyear & Nelson, 1997). Haggerty and Hilsenroth (2011) described this challenge:

> Suppose a loved one has to undergo surgery and you need to choose between two surgeons, one of whom has never been directly observed by an experienced surgeon while performing any surgery. He or she would perform the surgery and return to his or her attending physician and try to recall, sometimes incompletely or inaccurately, the intricate steps of the surgery they just performed. It is hard to imagine that anyone, given a choice, would prefer this over a professional who has been routinely observed in the practice of their craft. (p. 193)

Criterion 2: Provide Continual Corrective Feedback

Trainees need corrective feedback to learn what they are doing well, what they are doing poorly, and how to improve their skills. Feedback should be as specific and incremental as possible. Following are examples of specific feedback: "Your voice sounds rushed. Try slowing down by pausing for a few seconds between your statements to the client" and "You're doing an excellent job at making eye contact with the client." Examples of vague and nonspecific feedback are as follows: "Try to build better rapport with the client" and "Try to be more open to the client's feelings."

Criterion 3: Specific Skill Rehearsal Just Beyond the Trainees' Current Ability (Zone of Proximal Development)

Deliberate practice emphasizes skill acquisition via behavioral rehearsal. Trainers should endeavor not to get caught up in client conceptualization at the expense of focusing on skills. For many trainers, this requires significant discipline and self-restraint. It is simply more enjoyable to talk about psychotherapy theory (e.g., case conceptualization, treatment planning, nuances of psychotherapy models, similar cases the supervisor has had) than watch trainees rehearse skills. Trainees have many questions, and supervisors have an abundance of experience; the allotted supervision time can easily be filled by sharing knowledge. The supervisor gets to sound smart, while the trainee doesn't have to struggle with acquiring skills at their learning edge. Although answering questions is important, trainees' intellectual knowledge about psychotherapy can quickly surpass their procedural ability to perform psychotherapy, particularly with clients they find challenging. Here's a simple rule of thumb: The trainer provides the knowledge, but the behavioral rehearsal provides the skill (Rousmaniere, 2019).

Criterion 4: Practice at the Right Difficulty Level (Neither Too Easy nor Too Challenging)

Deliberate practice involves *optimal strain*: practicing skills just beyond the trainee's current skill threshold so that they can learn incrementally without becoming overwhelmed (Ericsson, 2006).

Trainers should use difficulty assessments and adjustments throughout deliberate practice to ensure that trainees are practicing at the right difficulty level. Note that some trainees are surprised by their unpleasant reactions to exercises (e.g., dissociation, nausea, blanking out), and may be tempted to "push through" exercises that are too hard. This can happen out of fear of failing a course, fear of being judged as incompetent, or negative self-impressions by the trainee (e.g., "This shouldn't be so hard"). Trainers should normalize the fact that there will be wide variation in perceived difficulty of the exercises and encourage trainees to respect their own personal training process.

Criterion 5: Continuously Assess Trainee Performance With Real Clients

The goal of deliberately practicing psychotherapy skills is to improve trainees' effectiveness at helping real clients. One of the risks in deliberate practice training is that the benefits will not generalize: Trainees' acquired competence in specific skills may not translate into work with real clients. Thus, it is important that trainers assess the impact of deliberate practice on trainees' work with real clients. Ideally, this is done through triangulation of multiple data points:

- client data (verbal self-report and routine outcome monitoring data)
- supervisor's report
- trainee's self-report

If the trainee's effectiveness with real clients is not improving after deliberate practice, the trainer should do a careful assessment of the difficulty. If the supervisor or trainer feels it is a skill acquisition issues, they may want to consider adjusting the deliberate practice routine to better suit the trainee's learning needs or style.

Therapists have traditionally been evaluated from a lens of *process accountability* (Markman & Tetlock, 2000; see also Goodyear, 2015), which focuses on demonstrating specific behaviors (e.g., fidelity to a treatment model) without regard to the impact on clients. We propose that clinical effectiveness is better assessed through a lens tightly focused on client outcomes and that learning objectives shift from performing behaviors that experts have decided are effective (i.e., the competence model) to highly individualized behavioral goals tailored to each trainee's zone of proximal development and performance feedback. This model of assessment has been termed *outcome accountability* (Goodyear, 2015), which focuses on client changes, rather than therapist competence, independent of how the therapist might be performing expected tasks.

Guidance for Trainees

The central theme of this book has been that skill rehearsal is not automatically helpful. Deliberate practice must be done well for trainees to benefit (Ericsson & Pool, 2016). In this chapter and in the exercises, we offer guidance for effective deliberate practice. We would also like to provide additional advice specifically for trainees. That advice is drawn from what we have learned at our volunteer deliberate practice test sites around the world. We cover how to discover your own training process, active effort, playfulness and taking breaks during deliberate practice, your right to control your self-disclosure to trainers, monitoring training results, monitoring complex reactions toward the trainer, and your own personal therapy.

Individualized IPT Training: Finding Your Zone of Proximal Development

Deliberate practice works best when training targets each trainee's personal skill thresholds. Also termed the *zone of proximal development*, a term first coined by Vygotsky in reference to developmental learning theory (Zaretskii, 2009), this is the area just beyond the trainee's current ability but that is possible to reach with the assistance of a teacher or coach (Wass & Golding, 2014). **If a deliberate practice exercise is either too easy or too hard, the trainee will not benefit.** To maximize training productivity, elite performers follow a "challenging but not overwhelming" principle: Tasks that are too far beyond their capacity will prove ineffective and even harmful, and it is equally true that mindlessly repeating what they can already do confidently will prove fruitless. Because of this, deliberate practice requires ongoing assessment of the trainee's current skill and concurrent difficulty adjustment to target a "good enough" challenge consistently. Thus, if you are practicing Exercise 5 ("Helping the Client to Describe Their Distress and Need for Support"), and it just feels too difficult, consider moving back to a more comfortable skill such as Exercise 4 ("Interpersonal Framing of Distress") or Exercise 3 ("Clarifications") that they may feel they have already mastered.

Active Effort

It is important for trainees to maintain an active and sustained effort, while doing the deliberate practice exercises in this book. Deliberate practice really helps when trainees push themselves up to and past their current ability. This is best achieved when trainees take ownership of their own practice by guiding their training partners to adjust role-plays to be as high on the difficulty scale as possible without hurting themselves. This will look different for every trainee. Although it can feel uncomfortable or even frightening, this is the zone of proximal development where the most gains can be made. Simply reading and repeating the written scripts will provide little or no benefit. Trainees are advised to remember that their effort from training should lead to more confidence and comfort in session with real clients.

Stay the Course: Effort Versus Flow

The deliberate practice only works if trainees push themselves hard enough to break out of their old patterns of performance, which then permits growth of new skills (Ericsson & Pool, 2016). Because deliberate practice constantly focuses on the current edge of one's performance capacity, it is inevitably a straining endeavor. Indeed, professionals are unlikely to make lasting performance improvements unless there is sufficient engagement in tasks that are just at the edge of one's current capacity (Ericsson, 2003,

2006). From athletics or fitness training, many of us are familiar with this process of being pushed out of our comfort zones followed by adaptation. The same process applies to our mental and emotional abilities.

Many trainees might be surprised to discover that deliberate practice for IPT feels harder than psychotherapy with a real client. This may be because when working with a real client a therapist can get into a state of *flow* (Csikszentmihalyi, 1997), where work feels effortless. As young IPT therapists in training, clinicians are instructed to maintain the conceptual focus on interpersonal aspects of clients' presentations. Specifically, when asking questions or making clarifications, IPT clinicians are asked to focus on interpersonal functioning to expand clients' interpersonal awareness. This might be challenging to maintain throughout the session because, for some clinicians, this might be a new way to look at the content and process in therapy. Sometimes clinicians who are new to IPT might find it difficult to continue to hold conceptual focus on interpersonal distress. In such cases, therapists may want to move back to offering response formats with which they are more familiar and feel more proficient and try those for a short time, in part to increase a sense of confidence and mastery.

Discover Your Own Training Process

The effectiveness of deliberate practice is directly related to the effort and ownership trainees exert while doing the exercises. Trainers can provide guidance, but it is important for trainees to learn about their own idiosyncratic training processes over time. This will let them become masters of their own training and prepare for a career-long process of professional development. The following are a few examples of personal training processes trainees discovered while engaging in deliberate practice:

- One trainee noticed that she needed to master and understand, more than other clinicians, the initial examples in each exercise before she was to be able to move on and start practicing an exercise on her own.

- One trainee noticed that she needed to go back to Chapter 1 to catch the "therapeutic stance and spirit" of IPT, before she could start practicing exercises.

- One trainee noticed that she was good at persisting when an exercise is challenging but also that she requires more rehearsal than other trainees to feel comfortable with a new skill. This trainee focused on developing patience with her own pace of progress.

- One trainee noticed that he could acquire new skills rather quickly, with only a few repetitions. However, he also noticed that his reactions to evocative client statements could jump very quickly and unpredictably from the "good challenge" to the "too hard" categories, so he needed to attend carefully to the reactions listed on the Deliberate Practice Reaction Form.

- One trainee described herself as "perfectionistic" and felt a strong urge to "push through" an exercise even when she had anxiety reactions, such as nausea and dissociation, in the "too hard" category. This caused the trainee not to benefit from the exercises and risk becoming demoralized. This trainee focused on going slower, developing self-compassion regarding her anxiety reactions, and asking her training partners to make role-plays less challenging.

Trainees are encouraged to reflect deeply on their own experiences using the exercises to learn the most about themselves and their personal learning processes.

Playfulness and Taking Breaks

Psychotherapy is serious work that often involves painful feelings. However, practicing psychotherapy can be playful and fun (Scott Miller, personal communication, 2017). Trainees should remember that one of the main goals of deliberate practice is to experiment with different approaches and styles of therapy. If deliberate practice ever feels rote, boring, or routine, it probably isn't going to help advance trainees' skill. In this case, trainees should try to liven it up. A good way to do this is to introduce an atmosphere of playfulness. For example, trainees can try the following:

- Use different vocal tones, speech pacing, body gestures, or other languages. This can expand trainees' communication range.

- Practice while simulating being blind (with a blindfold). This can increase sensitivity in the other senses.

- Practice while standing up or walking around outside. This can help trainees get new perspectives on the process of therapy.

The supervisor can also ask trainees if they would like to take a 5- to 10-minute break between questions, particularly if the trainees are dealing with difficult emotions and are feeling stressed out.

Additional Deliberate Practice Opportunities

This book focuses on deliberate practice methods that involve active, live engagement between trainees and a supervisor. Importantly, deliberate practice can extend beyond these focused training sessions as be used for homework. For example, a trainee might read the client stimuli quietly or aloud and practice their responses independently between sessions with a supervisor. In such cases, it is important for the trainee to say their therapist responses aloud, rather than rehearse silently in one's head. Alternatively, two trainees can practice as a pair, without the supervisor. Although the absence of a supervisor limits one source of feedback, the peer trainee who is playing the client can serve this role, as they can when a supervisor is present. These additional deliberate practice opportunities are intended to take place between focused training sessions with a supervisor. To optimize the quality of the deliberate practice when conducted independently or without a supervisor, we have developed a Deliberate Practice Diary Form that can be found in Appendix B or downloaded from https://www.apa.org/pubs/books/deliberate-practice-interpersonal-psychotherapy (see the "Resources" tab). This form provides a template for the trainee to record their experience of the deliberate practice activity, and, ideally, it will aid in the consolidation of learning. This form can be used as part of the evaluation process with the supervisor but is not necessarily intended for that purpose, and trainees are certainly welcome to bring their experience with the independent practice into the next meeting with the supervisor.

Monitoring Training Results

While trainers will evaluate trainees using a competency-focused model, trainees are also encouraged to take ownership of their own training process and look for results of deliberate practice themselves. Trainees should experience the results of deliberate practice within a few training sessions. A lack of results can be demoralizing for trainees and can result in their applying less effort and focus in deliberate practice. Trainees who are not seeing results should openly discuss this problem with their trainer and experiment with adjusting their deliberate practice process. Results can include client outcomes and improving the trainee's own work as a therapist, their personal development, and their overall training.

Client Outcomes

The most important result of deliberate practice is an improvement in trainees' client outcomes. This can be assessed via routine outcome measurement (Lambert, 2010; Prescott et al., 2017), qualitative data (McLeod, 2017), and informal discussions with clients. However, trainees should note that an improvement in client outcome due to deliberate practice can sometimes be challenging to achieve quickly, given that the largest amount of variance in client outcome is due to client variables (Bohart & Wade, 2013). For example, a client with severe chronic symptoms may not respond quickly to any treatment, regardless of how effectively a trainee practices. For some clients, an increase in patience and self-compassion regarding their symptoms may be a sign of progress, rather than an immediate decrease in symptoms. Thus, trainees are advised to keep their expectations for client change realistic in the context of their client's symptoms, history, and presentation. It is important that trainees do not try to force their clients to improve in therapy for the trainee to feel like they are making progress in their training (Rousmaniere, 2016).

Trainee's Work as a Therapist

One important result of deliberate practice is change within the trainee regarding their work with clients. For example, trainees at test sites reported feeling more comfortable sitting with evocative clients, more confident addressing uncomfortable topics in therapy, and more responsive to a broader range of clients.

Trainee's Personal Development

Another important result of deliberate practice is personal growth within the trainee. For example, trainees at test sites reported becoming more in touch with their own feelings, increased self-compassion, and enhanced motivation to work with a broader range of clients.

Trainee's Training Process

Another valuable result of deliberate practice is improvement in the trainees' training process. For example, trainees at test sites reported becoming more aware of their personal training style, preferences, strengths, and challenges. Over time, trainees should grow to feel more ownership of their training process. Training to become a psychotherapist is a complex process that occurs over many years. Experienced, expert therapists still report continuing to grow well beyond their graduate school years (Orlinsky et al., 2005). Furthermore, training is not a linear process. Some clinicians reported feeling "good enough mastery" of the IPT approach after implementing it with two or three clients, from the beginning to the very end of treatment.

The Trainee–Trainer Alliance: Monitoring Complex Reactions Toward the Trainer

Trainees who engage in hard deliberate practice often report experiencing complex feelings toward their trainer. For example, one trainee said, "I know this is helping, but I also don't look forward to it!" Another trainee reported feeling both appreciation and frustration toward her trainer simultaneously. Trainees are advised to remember intensive training they have done in other fields, such as athletics or music. When a coach pushes a trainee to the edge of their ability, it is common for trainees to have complex reactions toward them.

This does not necessarily mean that the trainer is doing anything wrong. In fact, intensive training inevitably stirs up reactions toward the trainer, such as frustration, annoyance, disappointment, or anger, that coexist with the appreciation they feel. In fact, if trainees do not experience complex reactions, it is worth considering if the deliberate practice is sufficiently challenging. But what we asserted earlier about rights to privacy apply here as well. Because professional mental health training is hierarchical, and evaluative, trainers should not require or even expect trainees to share complex reactions they may be experiencing toward them. Trainers should stay open to their sharing, but the choice always remains with the trainee.

Trainee's Own Therapy

When engaging in deliberate practice, many trainees discover aspects of their inner world that may benefit from attending their own psychotherapy. For example, one trainee discovered that her clients' anger stirred up her own painful memories of abuse, another trainee found himself disassociating while practicing empathy skills, and another trainee experienced overwhelming shame and self-judgment when she couldn't master skills after just a few repetitions.

Although these discoveries were unnerving at first, they ultimately were very beneficial because they motivated the trainees to seek out their own therapy. Many therapists attend their own therapy. In fact, Norcross and Guy (2005) found in their review of 17 studies that about 75% of the more than 8,000 therapist participants have attended their own therapy. Orlinsky et al. (2005) found that more than 90% of therapists who attended their own therapy reported it as helpful.

QUESTIONS FOR TRAINEES
1. Are you balancing the effort to improve your skills with patience and self-compassion for your learning process?
2. Are you attending to any shame or self-judgment that arising from training?
3. Are you being mindful of your personal boundaries and also respecting any complex feelings you may have toward your trainers?

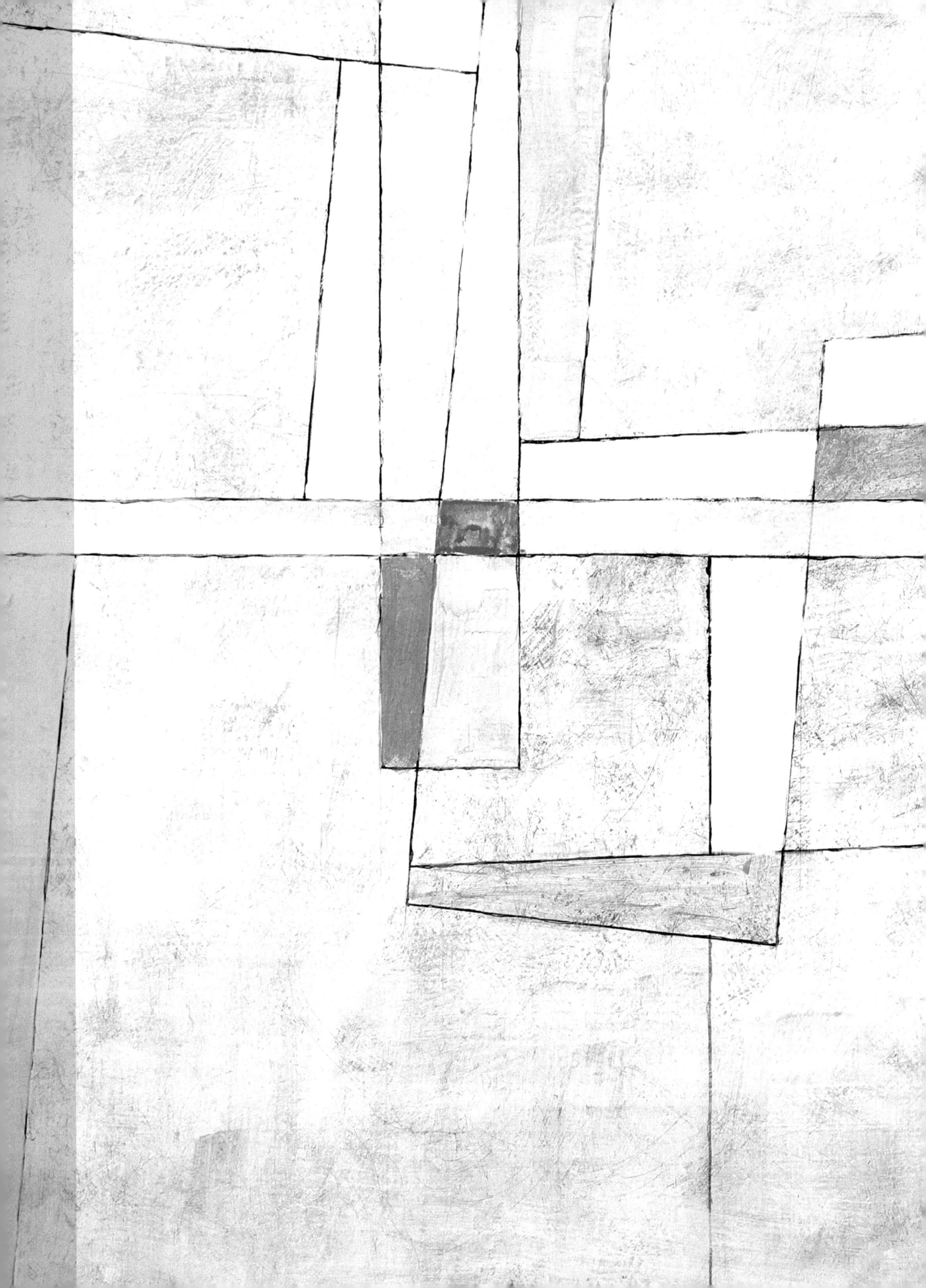

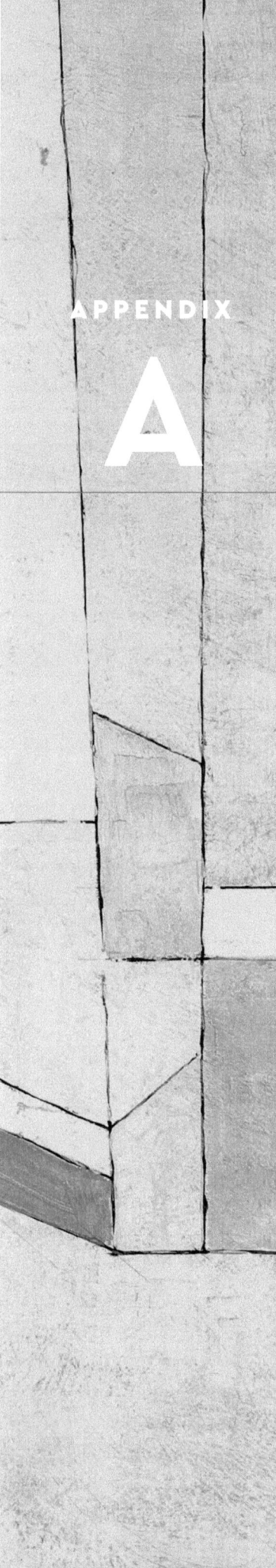

Difficulty Assessments and Adjustments

Deliberate practice works best if the exercises are performed at a good challenge that is neither too hard nor too easy. To ensure that they are practicing at the correct difficulty, trainees should do a difficulty assessment and adjustment after each level of client statement is completed (beginner, intermediate, and advanced). To do this, use the following instructions and the Deliberate Practice Reaction Form (Figure A.1), which is also available in the "Resources" tab online (https://www.apa.org/pubs/books/deliberate-practice-interpersonal-psychotherapy). **Do not skip this process!**

How to Assess Difficulty

The therapist completes the Deliberate Practice Reaction Form (Figure A.1). If they

- rate the difficulty of the exercise above an 8 or had any of the reactions in the "Too Hard" column, follow the instructions to make the exercise easier;

- rate the difficulty of the exercise below a 4 or didn't have any of the reactions in the "Good Challenge" column, proceed to the next level of harder client statements or follow the instructions to make exercise harder; or

- rate the difficulty of the exercise between 4 and 8 and have at least one reaction in the "Good Challenge" column, do not proceed to the harder client statements but rather repeat the same level.

Making Client Statements Easier

If the therapist ever rates the difficulty of the exercise above an 8 or has any of the reactions in the "Too Hard" column, use the next level easier client statements (e.g., if you were using advanced client statements, switch to intermediate). But if you already were using beginner client statements, use the following methods to make the client statements even easier:

- The person playing the client can use the same beginner client statements but this time in a softer, calmer voice and with a smile. This softens the emotional tone.

FIGURE A.1. Deliberate Practice Reaction Form

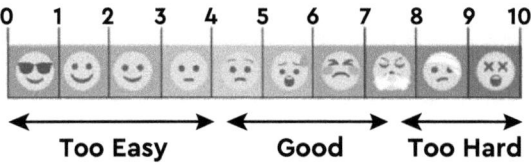

Question 1: How challenging was it to fulfill the skill criteria for this exercise?

Question 2: Did you have any reactions in "good challenge" or "too hard" categories? (yes/no)

Good Challenge			Too Hard		
Emotions and Thoughts	Body Reactions	Urges	Emotions and Thoughts	Body Reactions	Urges
Manageable shame, self-judgment, irritation, anger, sadness, etc.	Body tension, sighs, shallow breathing, increased heart rate, warmth, dry mouth	Looking away, withdrawing, changing focus	Severe or overwhelming shame, self-judgment, rage, grief, guilt, etc.	Migraines, dizziness, foggy thinking, diarrhea, disassociation, numbness, blanking out, nausea, etc.	Shutting down, giving up

Too Easy ⬇ Proceed to next difficulty level	Good Challenge ⬇ Repeat the same difficulty level	Too Hard ⬇ Go back to previous difficulty level

Note. From *Deliberate Practice in Emotion-Focused Therapy* (p. 180), by R. N. Goldman, A. Vaz, and T. Rousmaniere, 2021, American Psychological Association (https://doi.org/10.1037/0000227-000). Copyright 2021 by the American Psychological Association.

- The client can improvise with topics that are less evocative or make the therapist more comfortable, such as talking about topics without expressing feelings, the future or past (avoiding the here and now), or any topic outside therapy (see Figure A.2).

- The therapist can take a short break (5–10 minutes) between questions.

- The trainer can expand the "feedback phase" by discussing IPT or psychotherapy theory and research. This should shift the trainees' focus toward more detached or intellectual topics and reduce the emotional intensity.

Making Client Statements Harder

If the therapist rates the difficulty of the exercise below a 4 or didn't have any of the reactions in the "Good Challenge" column, proceed to next level harder client statements. If you were already using the advanced client statements, the client should make the exercise even harder, using the following guidelines:

- The person playing the client can use the advanced client statements again with a more distressed voice (e.g., very angry, sad, sarcastic) or unpleasant facial expression. This should increase the emotional tone.

FIGURE A.2. How to Make Client Statements Easier or Harder in Role-Plays

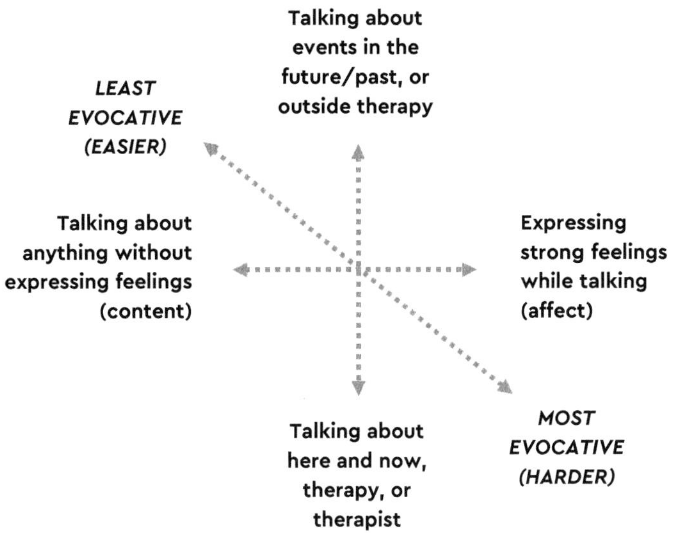

Note. Figure created by Jason Whipple, PhD.

- The client can improvise new client statements with topics that are more evocative or make the therapist uncomfortable, such as expressing strong feelings or talking about the here and now, therapy, or the therapist (see Figure A.2).

Note. The purpose of a deliberate practice session is not to get through all the client statements and therapist responses, but rather to spend as much time as possible practicing at the correct difficulty level. This may mean that trainees repeat the same statements/responses many times, which is okay, as long as the difficulty remains at the "Good Challenge" level.

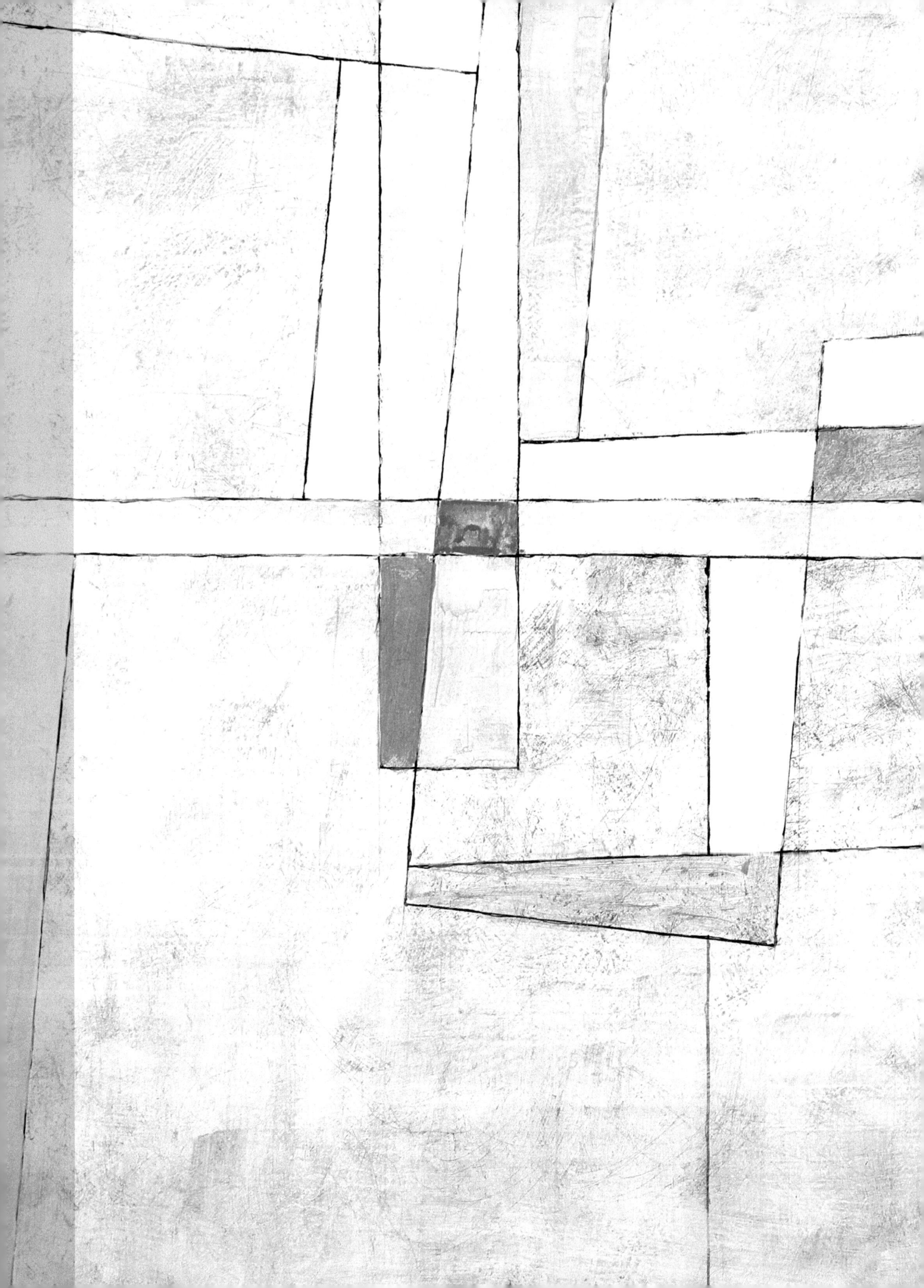

Deliberate Practice Diary Form

This book focuses on deliberate practice methods that involve active, live engagement between trainees and a supervisor. Importantly, deliberate practice can extend beyond these focused training sessions. For example, a trainee might read the client stimuli quietly or aloud and practice their responses independently between sessions with a supervisor. In such cases, it is important for the trainee to speak aloud rather than rehearse silently in one's head. Alternatively, two trainees can practice without the supervisor. Although the absence of a supervisor limits one source of feedback, the peer trainee who is playing the client can serve this role, as they can when a supervisor is present. Importantly, these additional deliberate practice opportunities are intended to take place between focused training sessions with a supervisor. To optimize the quality of the deliberate practice when conducted independently or without a supervisor, we have developed a Deliberate Practice Diary Form that can also be downloaded from the "Resources" tab online (https://www.apa.org/pubs/books/deliberate-practice-interpersonal-psychotherapy). This form provides a template for the trainee to record their experience of the deliberate practice activity and, ideally, will aid in the consolidation of learning. This form can also be used as part of the evaluation process with the supervisor but is not necessarily intended for that purpose, and trainees are certainly welcome to bring their experience with the independent practice into the next meeting with the supervisor.

Deliberate Practice Diary Form

Use this form to consolidate learnings from the deliberate practice exercises. Please protect your personal boundaries by only sharing information that you are comfortable disclosing.

Name: _____ Date: _____
Exercise: _____

Question 1. What was helpful or worked well this deliberate practice session? In what way?

Question 2. What was unhelpful or didn't go well this deliberate practice session? In what way?

Question 3. What did you learn about yourself, your current skills, and skills you'd like to keep improving? Feel free to share any details, but only those you are comfortable disclosing.

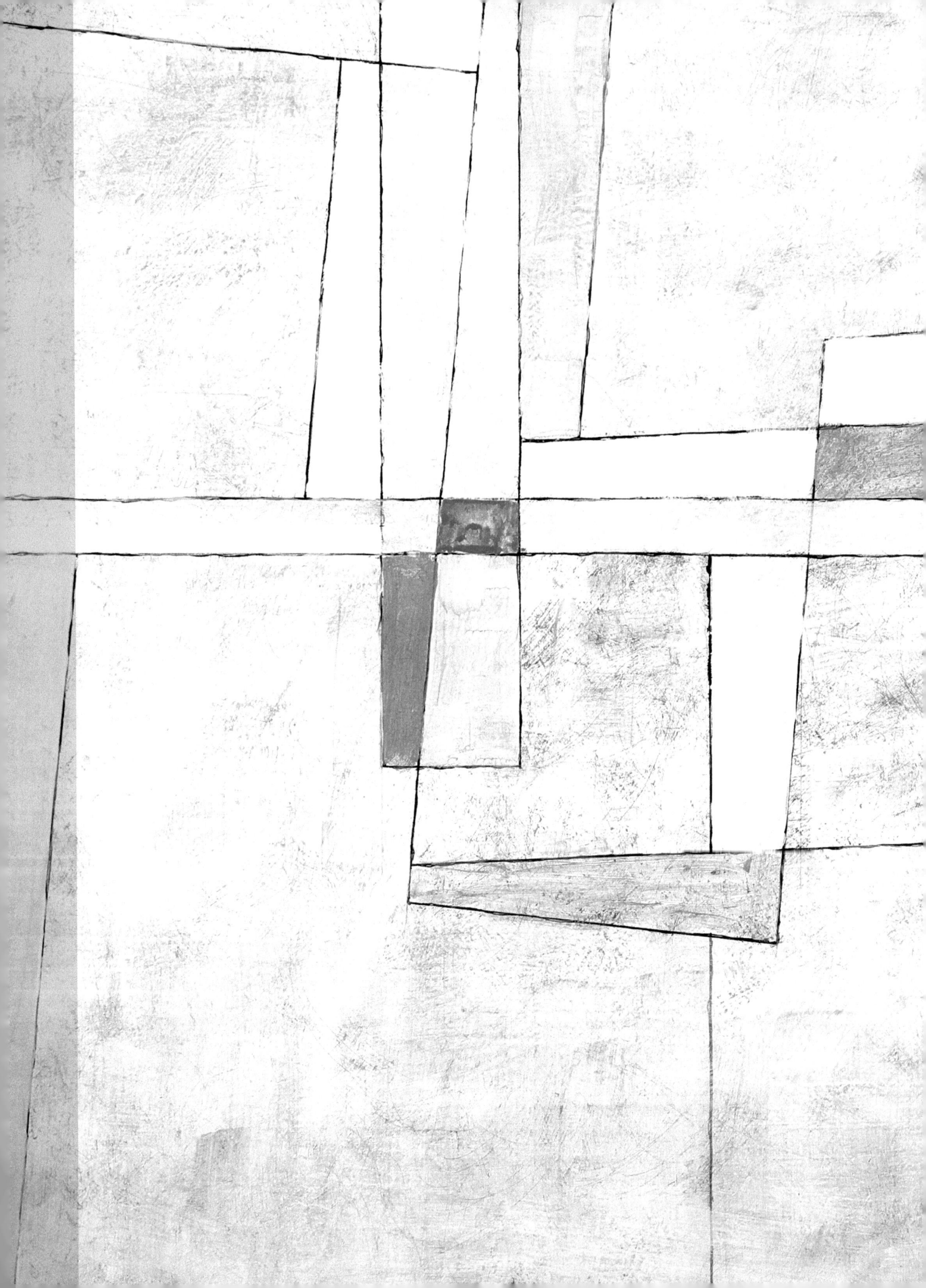

Additional Approaches and Troubleshooting When Implementing the Interpersonal Inventory

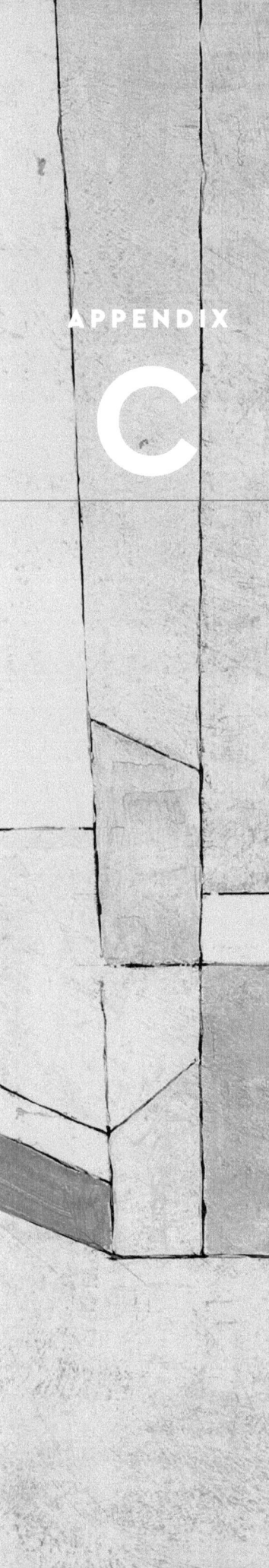

When implementing Interpersonal Inventory II (Exercise 2), clinicians can use a couple of approaches.

Approach 1

After the introduction of Exercise 1, "Presenting the Interpersonal Inventory," clinicians can ask the client some general questions about their experience of completing the inventory. Clinicians can also ask general questions about interpersonal dynamics with people in the Circle. Here are examples of some of the questions clinicians can ask the client:

1. How was this experience of completing the Interpersonal Inventory for you?

2. Did you have anyone in mind that you were going to place in one of the circles but ended up not writing down their name?

3. Did you end up placing someone in one of the circles and was surprised that they "made it in"?

4. What are the similarities and differences between people who are in the "intimate," "close," and "extended" support circles?
   a. What does it take to be in your "intimate" support, and what does it take to move out from "intimate" to "close" to "extended" support?
      i. Clinician can ask for examples that support the answers to these questions

5. Is everyone on the Circle exactly where you want them to be? Do you have someone who is too close, and you wish they were further away? Do you have someone who is too far away from you, and you wish they were closer to you?
   a. Clinicians can ask the client to draw arrows from the person to the space in the Interpersonal Inventory where the client ultimately wants them to be.

6. Who on this inventory understands you the most?
   a. What is it about them and you that allows for that understanding to occur?

7. Who in this inventory understands you the least?
   a. What is it about them and you that allows for that lack of understanding to occur?

8. If you are working with interpersonal disputes as a problem area, you can ask: Who is the easiest to disagree with, and what is it about them and you that allows for that to occur?

9. After discussing the experience of completing the Interpersonal Inventory and following up with some general questions, we can start asking questions specific to different people on the Circle.

Approach 2

The clinician can start Part 2 by asking the client right away about specific people on their Interpersonal Inventory:

1. Tell me a story about one of the people on the Circle.
2. What kind of emotional support do you get from Chris?
3. What kinds of support would you like to get from Chris?
4. What is it like for you to ask for help from Chris?
5. How well do you feel understood by Chris?
6. What do you wish you could change in your relationship with Chris?
7. What happens between the two of you when you disagree?
8. What do you typically disagree about, and how do you usually resolve it?
9. Have you ever told Chris about your current situation—your struggles, your needs, and your feelings?
10. How often do you see Chris?
11. How have your current symptoms impacted your relationship with Chris?

Troubleshooting When Implementing the Interpersonal Inventory

Question 1

What if the client puts the clinician on the Interpersonal Inventory?

Answer

When the client indicates the clinician's importance and places them in their Circle, the clinician works to understand what allowed the client to place the clinician in their Circle. For example, the clinician can ask the following questions to gain additional understanding:

1. What is it about our relationship that works for you?
    a. What aspect of our relationship resonates with you?
2. What is it about me or my way of relating with or to you that seems to work for you?
3. Who else in your life has or had similar characteristics?

The clinician can further highlight that the same qualities could be found in other people; the clinician can also inquire if the identified qualities and aspects of the relationship fall under the relational values for the client (e.g., honesty, directness). This knowledge could assist the client in further extending their social support with the intentionality of selecting people and relationships who match the client's values.

Question 2

What if the client does not have a lot of social support or puts in just two or three people?

Answer

If the client does not have a lot of social support in their Circle, the clinician can further explore how their current social support works and does not work for them. For example, the following questions could be asked:

1. In what way does your current social support work and not work for you?
2. Given your current social support, what type of support would you like to add to your Circle?

At the end of the discussion, if the client is interested in expanding their current social support, the clinician can inquire if this could be one of the aspects or goals to focus on in treatment.

Question 3

What if the client puts themselves into the Interpersonal Inventory?

Answer

If the client places themselves in the Circle, ask some questions about the relationship that the client has with themselves.

Question 4

What if the client has a lot of people to place, say 20 or 30?

Answer

When the client places a lot of people on a circle, the clinician can narrow down the discussion by asking the following questions:

1. Out of all the people in the circles, who do you feel might be helpful to discuss today?
2. Who occupies your mind the most at this time?

The clinician can direct the client to choose seven to nine people and indicate that as the sessions go by, they will discuss other people as they come up.

Question 5

Can clients place their pets or people who passed away in the Circle?

Answer

Yes, you can indicate to the client that they can place in the Circle someone who has passed away, their pets, and groups of people (e.g., a church or spiritual community, volleyball team).

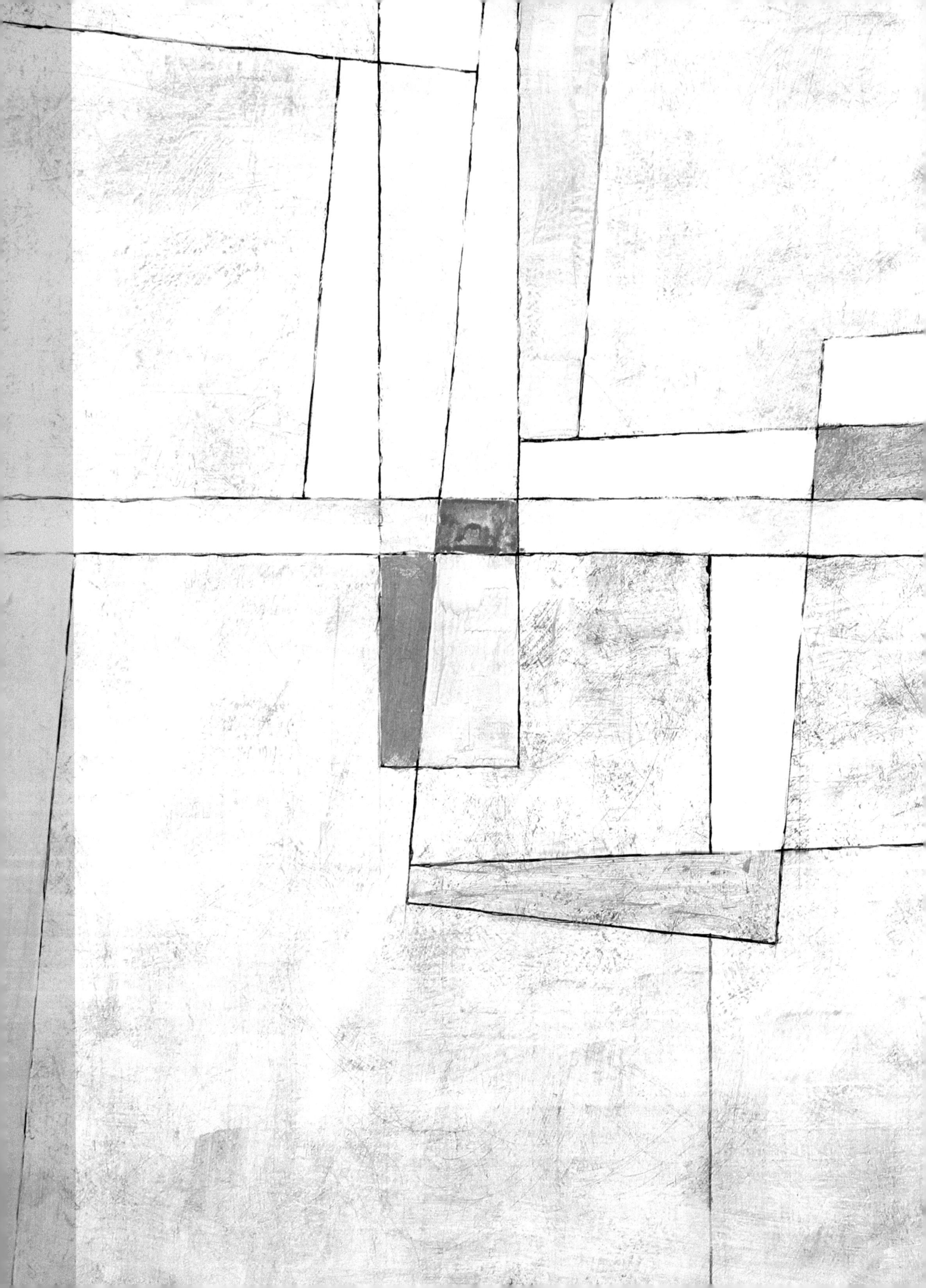

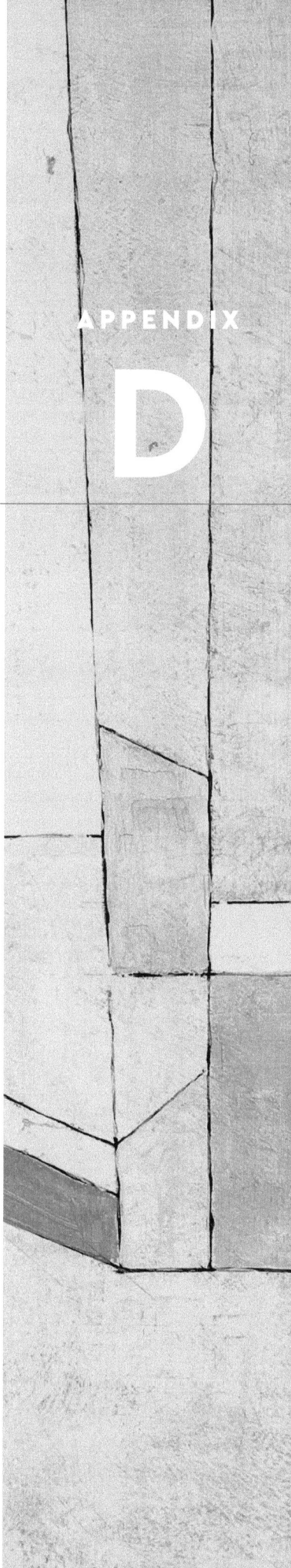

Sample Interpersonal Psychotherapy Syllabus With Embedded Deliberate Practice Exercises

This appendix provides a sample one-semester, three-unit course dedicated to teaching interpersonal psychotherapy (IPT). This course is appropriate for graduate students (master's and doctoral) at all levels of training, including first-year students who have not yet worked with clients. We present it as a model that can be adapted to a specific program's contexts and needs. For example, instructors may borrow portions of it to use in other courses, in practica, in didactic training events at externships and internships, in workshops, and in continuing education for postgraduate therapists.

Course Title: Interpersonal Psychotherapy: Theory and Deliberate Practice

Course Description

This course teaches theory, principles, and core skills of IPT. As a course with both didactic and practicum elements, it will review the theory and research on IPT and foster the use of deliberate practice to enable students to acquire 10 key IPT skills.

Course Objectives

Students who complete this course will be able to

1. describe the core theory, research, and skills of IPT.
2. apply the principles of deliberate practice for career-long clinical skill development.
3. demonstrate key IPT skills.
4. evaluate how they can fit IPT skills into their developing therapeutic framework.
5. employ IPT with clients from diverse cultural backgrounds.
6. describe the ways in which IPT is an evidenced-based practice.

Date	Lecture and Discussion	Skills Lab	Homework (for next class)
Week 1	Introduction to interpersonal psychotherapy (IPT): history and treatment overview	Exercise 1: Presenting the Interpersonal Inventory: Interpersonal Inventory I	Exercise 1; Markowitz & Weissman (2012); Stuart & Robertson (2012, Chapter 5); Stuart et al. (2017, in press); Weissman (2006)
Week 2	Theoretical basis for IPT: attachment and interpersonal theories	Repeat Exercise 1; Exercise 2: Exploring interpersonal relationships: Interpersonal Inventory II	Exercises 1 & 2; Ravitz et al. (2008); Stuart & Robertson (2012, Chapter 2)
Week 3	Effectiveness of IPT and IPT therapeutic stance	Exercise 3: Clarifications	Exercise 3; Cuijpers et al. (2011, 2016); Markowitz et al. (2014); Ravitz et al. (2019); Stuart & Robertson (2012, Chapter 8)
Week 4	Patient selection and IPT case conceptualization	Exercise 4: Interpersonal framing of distress	Exercise 4; Stuart & Robertson (2012, Chapters 4 & 6)
Week 5	IPT initial phase and treatment goals	Repeat Exercises 1 & 2	Exercises 1 & 2; Stuart & Robertson (2012, Chapter 3 & 7)
Week 6	IPT problem areas and middle phase of treatment	Exercise 5: Helping the client describe their distress and need for support	Exercise 5; Stuart & Robertson (2012, Chapters 14–16)
Week 7	Using communication analysis to understand communication	Exercise 7: Communication analysis	Exercise 7; Stuart & Robertson (2012, Chapter 9)
Week 8	Midterm paper due, self-evaluation, skill coaching feedback	Transcript session (Exercise 11) or mock session (Exercise 12) with a beginner client profile	Reading and exercise identified by mock or real session
Week 9	IPT techniques for working with communication and affect	Repeat Exercise 5; Exercise 6: Reinforcement of effective communication	Exercises 5 & 6; Stuart & Robertson (2012, Chapter 11); Weissman et al. (2018, Chapter 10)
Week 10	IPT techniques for improving communication	Exercise 8: Generating communication options	Exercise 8; Stuart & Robertson (2012, Chapters 10 & 12)
Week 11	IPT techniques for increasing social support	Exercise 9: Mobilizing social support	Exercise 9; Stuart & Robertson (2012, Chapters 2 & 13)
Week 12	IPT techniques for increasing social support	Exercise 10: Motivating interpersonal action	Exercise 10; Stuart & Robertson (2012, Chapter 13)
Week 13	Applications of IPT to diverse populations	Practice a mock session (Exercise 12) with an intermediate client profile	Cuijpers et al. (2018); Schultz & Stuart (2014); Stuart et al. (2021)
Week 14	IPT conclusion & maintenance phases	Practice a mock session (Exercise 12) with an advanced client profile	E. Frank et al. (2007); Stuart & Robertson (2012, Chapter 17)
Week 15	Final paper due, final exam, self-evaluation, skill coaching feedback	Transcript session (Exercise 11) or mock session (Exercise 12)	Reading and exercise identified by mock or real session

Format of Class

Classes are 3 hours long. Course time is split evenly between learning IPT theory and research and acquiring IPT skills.

Lecture/Discussion Class: Each week, there will be one Lecture/Discussion class for 1.5 hours focusing on IPT theory and related research.

IPT Skills Lab: Each week there will be one IPT Skills Lab for 1.5 hours. Skills Labs are for practicing IPT skills using the exercises in this book. The exercises use therapy simulations (role-plays) with the following goals:

1. Build trainees' abilities and confidence in using IPT skills with real clients.
2. Provide a safe space for experimenting with different therapeutic interventions, without fear of making mistakes.
3. Provide plenty of opportunity to explore and "try on" different styles of therapy, so trainees can ultimately discover their own personal, unique therapy style.

Mock Sessions: Twice during the semester (Weeks 8 and 15), trainees will do a psychotherapy mock session in the IPT skills lab. In contrast to highly structured and repetitive deliberate practice exercises, a psychotherapy mock session is an unstructured and improvised role-played therapy session. Mock sessions allow trainees to

1. practice using IPT skills responsively.
2. experiment with clinical decision making in an unscripted context.
3. discover their personal therapeutic style.
4. build endurance for working with real clients.

Homework

Homework will be assigned each week and will include reading, 1 hour of skills practice with an assigned practice partner, and occasional writing assignments. For the skills practice homework, trainees will repeat the exercise they did for that week's IPT skills lab. Because the instructor will not be there to evaluate performance, trainees should instead complete the Deliberate Practice Reaction Form, as well as the Deliberate Practice Diary Form, for themselves as a self-evaluation.

Writing Assignments

Students are to write two papers: one due at midterm and one due at the last day of class. Some possible topics for the papers are as follows:

- Exploration of one aspect of IPT theory, research, or technique
- A partial transcript of one of the trainees' therapy cases with a real client, with discussion from an IPT perspective

Multicultural Orientation

This course is taught in a multicultural context, defined as "how the cultural worldviews, values, and beliefs of the client and therapist interact and influence one another to cocreate a relational experience that is in the spirit of healing" (Davis et al., 2018, p. 3). Core features of the multicultural orientation include cultural comfort, humility, and responding to cultural opportunities (or previously missed opportunities). Throughout this course, students are encouraged to reflect on their own cultural identity and improve their ability to attune with their clients' cultural identities (Hook et al., 2017). For further guidance on this topic and deliberate practice exercises to improve multicultural skills, see the book *Deliberate Practice in Multicultural Therapy* (Harris et al., 2024).

Vulnerability, Privacy, and Boundaries

This course is aimed at developing IPT skills, self-awareness, and interpersonal skills in an experiential framework and as relevant to clinical work. This course is not psychotherapy or a substitute for psychotherapy. Students should interact at a level of self-disclosure that is personally comfortable and helpful to their own learning. Although becoming aware of internal emotional and psychological processes is necessary for a therapist's development, it is not necessary to reveal all that information to the trainer. It is important for students to sense their own level of safety and privacy. Students are not evaluated on the level of material that they choose to reveal in the class.

In accordance with the *Ethical Principles of Psychologists and Code of Conduct* (American Psychological Association, 2017), students are **not required to disclose personal information.** Because this class is about developing both interpersonal and IPT competence, following are some important points so that students are fully informed as they make choices to self-disclose:

- Students choose how much, when, and what to disclose. Students are not penalized for the choice not to share personal information.

- The learning environment is susceptible to group dynamics much like any other group space; therefore students may be asked to share their observations and experiences of the class environment with the singular goal of fostering a more inclusive and productive learning environment.

Confidentiality

To create a safe learning environment that is respectful of client and therapist information and diversity and to foster open and vulnerable conversation in class, students are required to agree to strict confidentiality within and outside of the instruction setting.

Evaluation

Self-Evaluation: At the end of the semester (Week 15), trainees will perform a self-evaluation. This will help trainees track their progress and identify areas for further development. The Guidance for Trainees section in Chapter 3 of this book highlights potential areas of focus for self-evaluation.

Grading Criteria

As designed, students would be accountable for the level and quality of their performance in the following:

- the discussion classes,
- the skills lab (exercises and mock sessions),
- homework,
- midterm and final papers, and
- a final exam.

Required Readings

Cuijpers, P., Donker, T., Weissman, M. M., Ravitz, P., & Cristea, I. A. (2016). Interpersonal psychotherapy for mental health problems: A comprehensive meta-analysis. *The American Journal of Psychiatry*, *173*(7), 680–687. https://doi.org/10.1176/appi.ajp.2015.15091141

Cuijpers, P., Geraedts, A. S., van Oppen, P., Andersson, G., Markowitz, J. C., & van Straten, A. (2011). Interpersonal psychotherapy for depression: A meta-analysis. *The American Journal of Psychiatry*, *168*(6), 581–592. https://doi.org/10.1176/appi.ajp.2010.10101411

Cuijpers, P., Karyotaki, E., Reijnders, M., Purgato, M., & Barbui, C. (2018). Psychotherapies for depression in low- and middle-income countries: A meta-analysis. *World Psychiatry*, *17*(1), 90–101. https://doi.org/10.1002/wps.20493

Frank, E., Kupfer, D. J., Buysse, D. J., Swartz, H. A., Pilkonis, P. A., Houck, P. R., Rucci, P., Novick, D. M., Grochocinski, V. J., & Stapf, D. M. (2007). Randomized trial of weekly, twice-monthly, and monthly interpersonal psychotherapy as maintenance treatment for women with recurrent depression. *The American Journal of Psychiatry*, *164*(5), 761–767. https://doi.org/10.1176/ajp.2007.164.5.761

Markowitz, J. C., Lipsitz, J., & Milrod, B. L. (2014). Critical review of outcome research on interpersonal psychotherapy for anxiety disorders. *Depression and Anxiety*, *31*(4), 316–325. https://doi.org/10.1002/da.22238

Markowitz, J. C., & Weissman, M. M. (2012). Interpersonal psychotherapy: Past, present and future. *Clinical Psychology & Psychotherapy*, *19*(2), 99–105. https://doi.org/10.1002/cpp.1774

Ravitz, P., Maunder, R., & McBride, C. (2008). Attachment, contemporary interpersonal theory and IPT: An integration of theoretical, clinical, and empirical perspectives. *Journal of Contemporary Psychotherapy*, *38*(1), 11–22. https://doi.org/10.1007/s10879-007-9064-y

Ravitz, P., Watson, P., Lawson, A., Constantino, M. J., Bernecker, S., Park, J., & Swartz, H. A. (2019). Interpersonal psychotherapy: A scoping review and historical perspective. *Harvard Review of Psychiatry*, *27*(3), 165–180. https://doi.org/10.1097/HRP.0000000000000219

Schultz, J. M., & Stuart, S. (2014). Interpersonal psychotherapy: A culturally adaptive treatment. *Psychotherapy in Australia*, *21*(1), 12–20.

Stuart, S., Pereira, X. V., & Chung, J. P. Y. (2021). Transcultural adaptation of interpersonal psychotherapy in Asia. *Asia-Pacific Psychiatry*, *13*(1), e12439. https://doi.org/10.1111/appy.12439

Stuart, S., & Robertson, M. (2012). *Interpersonal psychotherapy: A clinician's guide* (2nd ed.). Taylor & Francis.

Stuart, S., Schultz, J., Back-Price, A., Belik-Tuller, O., Stuart-Parrigon, K., Ashen, C., Fairhurst, S., Grause, A., & Brandon, A. (2017). *Interpersonal psychotherapy.* Scientific American Psychiatry.

Stuart, S., Schultz, J. M., Palmer Molina, A., & Siber-Sanderowitz, S. (in press). Interpersonal psychotherapy: A review of theory, history, and evidence of efficacy. *Psychodynamic Psychiatry*.

Weissman, M. (2006). A brief history of interpersonal psychotherapy. *Psychiatric Annals*, *36*(8), 553–557.

Weissman, M. M., Markowitz, J. C., & Klerman, G. L. (2018). *The guide to interpersonal psychotherapy* (Updated and expanded ed.). Oxford University Press.

Supplemental Readings

Elkin, I., Parloff, M. B., Hadley, S. W., & Autry, J. H. (1985). NIMH Treatment of Depression Collaborative Research Program. Background and research plan. *Archives of General Psychiatry*, *42*(3), 305–316. https://doi.org/10.1001/archpsyc.1985.01790260103013

Elkin, I., Shea, M. T., Watkins, J. T., Imber, S. D., Sotsky, S. M., Collins, F. L., Glass, D. R., Pilkonis, P. A., Leber, W. R., Doherty, J. P., Fiester, S. J., & Parloff, M. B. (1989). NIMH Treatment of Depression Collaborative Research Program: I. General effectiveness of treatments. *Archives of General Psychiatry*, *46*(11), 971–982. https://doi.org/10.1001/archpsyc.1989.01810110013002

Frank, E., Kupfer, D. J., Wagner, E. F., McEachran, A. B., & Cornes, C. (1991). Efficacy of interpersonal psychotherapy as a maintenance treatment of recurrent depression. Contributing factors.

Archives of General Psychiatry, 48(12), 1053–1059. https://doi.org/10.1001/archpsyc.1991.01810360017002

Klerman, G. L., & Weissman, M. M. (1993). *New applications of interpersonal psychotherapy.* American Psychiatric Press.

Klerman, G. L., Weissman, M. M., Rounsaville, B., & Chevron, E. S. (1984). *Interpersonal psychotherapy of depression.* Basic Books.

Markowitz, J. C. (2016). *Interpersonal psychotherapy for posttraumatic stress disorder.* Oxford University Press. https://doi.org/10.1093/med:psych/9780190465599.001.0001

McAlpine, R., & Hillin, A. (2021). *Interpersonal psychotherapy for adolescents: A clinician's guide.* Taylor & Francis.

Mufson, L. (2004). *Interpersonal psychotherapy for depressed adolescents* (2nd ed.). Guilford Press.

Stuart, S., & Schultz, J. (2015). *Interpersonal psychotherapy for groups clinician handbook.* IPT Institute.

Stuart, S., Schultz, J. M., & McCann, E. (2012). *Interpersonal psychotherapy: Clinician handbook.* IPT Institute Press.

Weissman, M., Markowitz, J. C., & Klerman, G. (2000). *Comprehensive guide to interpersonal psychotherapy.* Basic Books.

Wilfley, D. E., MacKenzie, K. R., Welch, R. R., Ayres, V. E., & Weissman, M. M. (2000). *Interpersonal psychotherapy for group.* Basic Books.

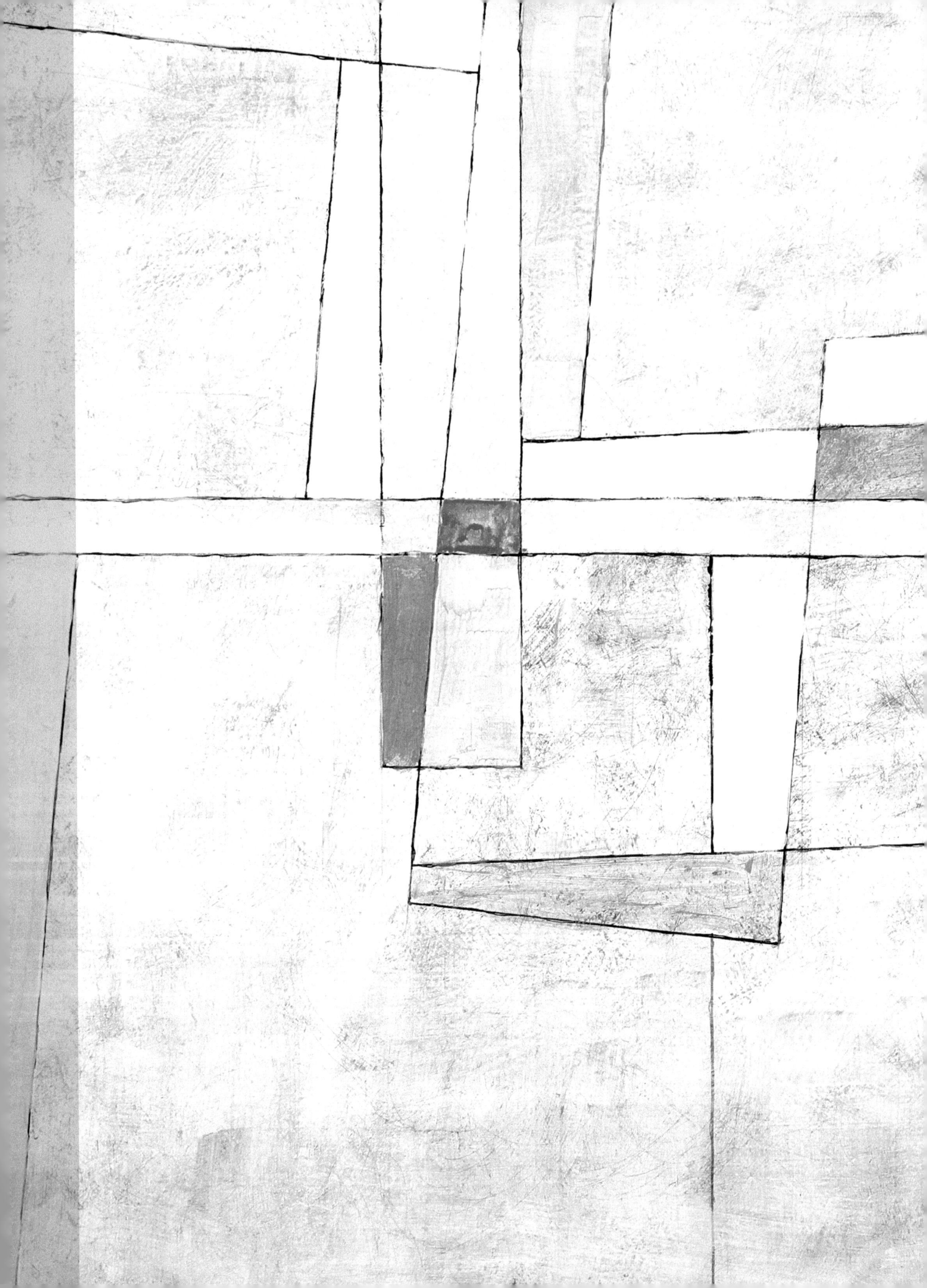

References

Althobaiti, S., Kazantzis, N., Ofori-Asenso, R., Romero, L., Fisher, J., Mills, K. E., & Liew, D. (2020). Efficacy of interpersonal psychotherapy for post-traumatic stress disorder: A systematic review and meta-analysis. *Journal of Affective Disorders, 264*, 286–294. https://doi.org/10.1016/j.jad.2019.12.021

American Psychological Association. (2017). *Ethical principles of psychologists and code of conduct* (2002, Amended June 1, 2010, and January 1, 2017). https://www.apa.org/ethics/code/

Anderson, T., Ogles, B. M., Patterson, C. L., Lambert, M. J., & Vermeersch, D. A. (2009). Therapist effects: Facilitative interpersonal skills as a predictor of therapist success. *Journal of Clinical Psychology, 65*(7), 755–768. https://doi.org/10.1002/jclp.20583

Bailey, R. J., & Ogles, B. M. (2019). Common factors as a therapeutic approach: What is required? *Practice Innovations, 4*(4), 241–254. https://doi.org/10.1037/pri0000100

Barlow, D. H. (2010). Negative effects from psychological treatments: A perspective. *American Psychologist, 65*(1), 13–20. https://doi.org/10.1037/a0015643

Barth, J., Munder, T., Gerger, H., Nüesch, E., Trelle, S., Znoj, H., Jüni, P., & Cuijpers, P. (2013). Comparative efficacy of seven psychotherapeutic interventions for patients with depression: A network meta-analysis. *PLOS Medicine, 10*(5), Article e1001454. https://doi.org/10.1371/journal.pmed.1001454

Bartholomew, K., & Horowitz, L. M. (1991). Attachment styles among young adults: A test of a four-category model. *Journal of Personality and Social Psychology, 61*(2), 226–244. https://doi.org/10.1037/0022-3514.61.2.226

Bass, J., Neugebauer, R., Clougherty, K. F., Verdeli, H., Wickramaratne, P., Ndogoni, L., Speelman, L., Weissman, M., & Bolton, P. (2006). Group interpersonal psychotherapy for depression in rural Uganda: 6-month outcomes: Randomised controlled trial. *The British Journal of Psychiatry, 188*(6), 567–573. https://doi.org/10.1192/bjp.188.6.567

Beck, A. T., Rush, A. J., Shaw, B. F., & Emery, G. (1979). *Cognitive therapy of depression*. Guilford Press.

Benjamin, L. S. (1996). *Interpersonal diagnosis and treatment of personality disorders* (2nd ed.). Guilford Press.

Bennett-Levy, J. (2019). Why therapists should walk the talk: The theoretical and empirical case for personal practice in therapist training and professional development. *Journal of Behavior Therapy and Experimental Psychiatry, 62*, 133–145. https://doi.org/10.1016/j.jbtep.2018.08.004

Bennett-Levy, J., & Finlay-Jones, A. (2018). The role of personal practice in therapist skill development: A model to guide therapists, educators, supervisors and researchers. *Cognitive Behaviour Therapy, 47*(3), 185–205. https://doi.org/10.1080/16506073.2018.1434678

Bohart, A. C., & Wade, A. G. (2013). The client in psychotherapy. In M. J. Lambert (Ed.), *Bergin and Garfield's handbook of psychotherapy and behavior change* (6th ed., 219–257). John Wiley & Sons.

Bolton, P., Bass, J., Neugebauer, R., Verdeli, H., Clougherty, K. F., Wickramaratne, P., Speelman, L., Ndogoni, L., & Weissman, M. (2003). Group interpersonal psychotherapy for depression in rural Uganda: A randomized controlled trial. *JAMA: Journal of the American Medical Association, 289*(23), 3117–3124. https://doi.org/10.1001/jama.289.23.3117

Bowlby, J. (1969). *Attachment and loss, Vol. 1: Attachment.* Basic Books.

Brandon, A. R., Ceccotti, N., Hynan, L. S., Shivakumar, G., Johnson, N., & Jarrett, R. B. (2012). Proof of concept: Partner-assisted interpersonal psychotherapy for perinatal depression. *Archives of Women's Mental Health, 15*(6), 469–480. https://doi.org/10.1007/s00737-012-0311-1

Bright, K. S., Charrois, E. M., Mughal, M. K., Wajid, A., McNeil, D., Stuart, S., Hayden, K. A., & Kingston, D. (2020). Interpersonal psychotherapy to reduce psychological distress in perinatal women: A systematic review. *International Journal of Environmental Research and Public Health, 17*(22), 8421. https://doi.org/10.3390/ijerph17228421

Bugatti, M., & Boswell, J. F. (2016). Clinical errors as a lack of context responsiveness. *Psychotherapy: Theory, Research, & Practice, 53*(3), 262–267. https://doi.org/10.1037/pst0000080

Castonguay, L. G., Goldfried, M. R., Wiser, S., Raue, P. J., & Hayes, A. M. (1996). Predicting the effect of cognitive therapy for depression: A study of unique and common factors. *Journal of Consulting and Clinical Psychology, 64*(3), 497–504. https://doi.org/10.1037/0022-006X.64.3.497

Coker, J. (1990). *How to practice jazz.* Jamey Aebersold.

Cook, R. (2005). *It's about that time: Miles Davis on and off record.* Atlantic Books.

Csikszentmihalyi, M. (1997). *Finding flow: The psychology of engagement with everyday life.* Harper Collins.

Cuijpers, P., Donker, T., Weissman, M. M., Ravitz, P., & Cristea, I. A. (2016). Interpersonal psychotherapy for mental health problems: A comprehensive meta-analysis. *The American Journal of Psychiatry, 173*(7), 680–687. https://doi.org/10.1176/appi.ajp.2015.15091141

Cuijpers, P., Geraedts, A. S., van Oppen, P., Andersson, G., Markowitz, J. C., & van Straten, A. (2011). Interpersonal psychotherapy for depression: A meta-analysis. *The American Journal of Psychiatry, 168*(6), 581–592. https://doi.org/10.1176/appi.ajp.2010.10101411

Cuijpers, P., Karyotaki, E., de Wit, L., & Ebert, D. D. (2020). The effects of fifteen evidence-supported therapies for adult depression: A meta-analytic review. *Psychotherapy Research, 30*(3), 279–293. https://doi.org/10.1080/10503307.2019.1649732

Cuijpers, P., Karyotaki, E., Reijnders, M., Purgato, M., & Barbui, C. (2018). Psychotherapies for depression in low- and middle-income countries: A meta-analysis. *World Psychiatry, 17*(1), 90–101. https://doi.org/10.1002/wps.20493

Cuijpers, P., Quero, S., Noma, H., Ciharova, M., Miguel, C., Karyotaki, E., Cipriani, A., Cristea, I. A., & Furukawa, T. A. (2021). Psychotherapies for depression: A network meta-analysis covering efficacy, acceptability and long-term outcomes of all main treatment types. *World Psychiatry, 20*(2), 283–293. https://doi.org/10.1002/wps.20860

Davis, D. E., DeBlaere, C., Owen, J., Hook, J. N., Rivera, D. P., Choe, E., Van Tongeren, D. R., Worthington, E. L., & Placeres, V. (2018). The multicultural orientation framework: A narrative review. *Psychotherapy: Theory, Research, & Practice, 55*(1), 89–100. https://doi.org/10.1037/pst0000160

Elkin, I., Shea, M. T., Watkins, J. T., Imber, S. D., Sotsky, S. M., Collins, F. L., Glass, D. R., Pilkonis, P. A., Leber, W. R., Doherty, J. P., Fiester, S. J., & Parloff, M. B. (1989). National Institute of Mental Health Treatment of Depression Collaborative Research Program: I. General effectiveness of treatments. *Archives of General Psychiatry, 46*(11), 971–982. https://doi.org/10.1001/archpsyc.1989.01810110013002

Ellis, M. V., Berger, L., Hanus, A. E., Ayala, E. E., Swords, B. A., & Siembor, M. (2014). Inadequate and harmful clinical supervision: Testing a revised framework and assessing occurrence. *The Counseling Psychologist, 42*(4), 434–472. https://doi.org/10.1177/0011000013508656

Ericsson, K. A. (2003). Development of elite performance and deliberate practice: An update from the perspective of the expert performance approach. In J. L. Starkes & K. A. Ericsson (Eds.), *Expert performance in sports: Advances in research on sport expertise* (pp. 49–83). Human Kinetics.

Ericsson, K. A. (2004). Deliberate practice and the acquisition and maintenance of expert performance in medicine and related domains: Invited address. *Academic Medicine, 79,* S70–S81. https://doi.org/10.1097/00001888-200410001-00022

Ericsson, K. A. (2006). The influence of experience and deliberate practice on the development of superior expert performance. In K. A. Ericsson, N. Charness, P. J. Feltovich, & R. R. Hoffman (Eds.), *The Cambridge handbook of expertise and expert performance* (pp. 683–704). Cambridge University Press. https://doi.org/10.1017/CBO9780511816796.038

Ericsson, K. A., Hoffman, R. R., Kozbelt, A., & Williams, A. M. (Eds.). (2018). *The Cambridge handbook of expertise and expert performance* (2nd ed.). Cambridge University Press. https://doi.org/10.1017/9781316480748

Ericsson, K. A., Krampe, R. T., & Tesch-Römer, C. (1993). The role of deliberate practice in the acquisition of expert performance. *Psychological Review, 100*(3), 363–406. https://doi.org/10.1037/0033-295X.100.3.363

Ericsson, K. A., & Pool, R. (2016). *Peak: Secrets from the new science of expertise.* Houghton Mifflin Harcourt.

Fairburn, C. G., Cooper, Z., & Shafran, R. (2003). Cognitive behaviour therapy for eating disorders: A "transdiagnostic" theory and treatment. *Behaviour Research and Therapy, 41*(5), 509–528. https://doi.org/10.1016/S0005-7967(02)00088-8

Fisher, R. P., & Craik, F. I. M. (1977). Interaction between encoding and retrieval operations in cued recall. *Journal of Experimental Psychology: Human Learning and Memory, 3*(6), 701–711. https://doi.org/10.1037/0278-7393.3.6.701

Frank, E., Kupfer, D. J., Buysse, D. J., Swartz, H. A., Pilkonis, P. A., Houck, P. R., Rucci, P., Novick, D. M., Grochocinski, V. J., & Stapf, D. M. (2007). Randomized trial of weekly, twice-monthly, and monthly interpersonal psychotherapy as maintenance treatment for women with recurrent depression. *The American Journal of Psychiatry, 164*(5), 761–767. https://doi.org/10.1176/ajp.2007.164.5.761

Frank, E., Kupfer, D. J., Perel, J. M., Cornes, C., Jarrett, D. B., Mallinger, A. G., Thase, M. E., McEachran, A. B., & Grochocinski, V. J. (1990). Three-year outcomes for maintenance therapies in recurrent depression. *Archives of General Psychiatry, 47*(12), 1093–1099. https://doi.org/10.1001/archpsyc.1990.01810240013002

Frank, E., Kupfer, D. J., Wagner, E. F., McEachran, A. B., & Cornes, C. (1991). Efficacy of interpersonal psychotherapy as a maintenance treatment of recurrent depression. Contributing factors. *Archives of General Psychiatry, 48*(12), 1053–1059. https://doi.org/10.1001/archpsyc.1991.01810360017002

Frank, J. D. (1971). Eleventh Emil A. Gutheil memorial conference. Therapeutic factors in psychotherapy. *American Journal of Psychotherapy, 25*(3), 350–361. https://doi.org/10.1176/appi.psychotherapy.1971.25.3.350

Gladwell, M. (2008). *Outliers: The story of success.* Little, Brown & Company.

Goldberg, S., Rousmaniere, T. G., Miller, S. D., Whipple, J., Nielsen, S. L., Hoyt, W., & Wampold, B. E. (2016). Do psychotherapists improve with time and experience? A longitudinal analysis of outcomes in a clinical setting. *Journal of Counseling Psychology, 63*(1), 1–11. https://doi.org/10.1037/cou0000131

Goldman, R. N., Vaz, A., & Rousmaniere, T. (2021). *Deliberate practice in emotion-focused therapy.* American Psychological Association. https://doi.org/10.1037/0000227-000

Goodyear, R. K. (2015). Using accountability mechanisms more intentionally: A framework and its implications for training professional psychologists. *American Psychologist, 70*(8), 736–743. https://doi.org/10.1037/a0039828

Goodyear, R. K., & Nelson, M. L. (1997). The major formats of psychotherapy supervision. In C. E. Watkins, Jr. (Ed.), *Handbook of psychotherapy supervision* (pp. 328–334). John Wiley & Sons.

Greenberg, L. S., & Goldman, R. L. (1988). Training in experiential therapy. *Journal of Consulting and Clinical Psychology, 56*(5), 696–702. https://doi.org/10.1037/0022-006X.56.5.696

Haggerty, G., & Hilsenroth, M. J. (2011). The use of video in psychotherapy supervision. *British Journal of Psychotherapy, 27*(2), 193–210. https://doi.org/10.1111/j.1752-0118.2011.01232.x

Harris, J., Jin, J., Hoffman, S., Phan, S., Prout, T. A., Rousmaniere, T., & Vaz, A. (2024). *Deliberate practice in multicultural therapy.* American Psychological Association. https://doi.org/10.1037/0000357-000

Hatcher, R. L. (2015). Interpersonal competencies: Responsiveness, technique, and training in psychotherapy. *American Psychologist, 70*(8), 747–757. https://doi.org/10.1037/a0039803

Henry, W. P., Strupp, H. H., Butler, S. F., Schacht, T. E., & Binder, J. L. (1993). Effects of training in time-limited dynamic psychotherapy: Changes in therapist behavior. *Journal of Consulting and Clinical Psychology, 61*(3), 434–440. https://doi.org/10.1037/0022-006X.61.3.434

Hill, C. E., Kivlighan, D. M. III, Rousmaniere, T., Kivlighan, D. M., Jr., Gerstenblith, J. A., & Hillman, J. W. (2020). Deliberate practice for the skill of immediacy: A multiple case study of doctoral student therapists and clients. *Psychotherapy, 57*(4), 587–597. https://doi.org/10.1037/pst0000247

Hill, C. E., & Knox, S. (2013). Training and supervision in psychotherapy: Evidence for effective practice. In M. J. Lambert (Ed.), *Handbook of psychotherapy and behavior change* (6th ed., pp. 775–811). John Wiley & Sons.

Hook, J. N., Davis, D. D., Owen, J., & DeBlaere, C. (2017). *Cultural humility: Engaging diverse identities in therapy.* American Psychological Association. https://doi.org/10.1037/0000037-000

Horowitz, L. M. (2004). *Interpersonal foundations of psychopathology.* American Psychological Association. https://doi.org/10.1037/10727-000

Johnson, J. E., Stout, R. L., Miller, T. R., Zlotnick, C., Cerbo, L. A., Andrade, J. T., Nargiso, J., Bonner, J., & Wiltsey-Stirman, S. (2019). Randomized cost-effectiveness trial of group interpersonal psychotherapy (IPT) for prisoners with major depression. *Journal of Consulting and Clinical Psychology, 87*(4), 392–406. https://doi.org/10.1037/ccp0000379

Kendall, P. C., & Beidas, R. S. (2007). Smoothing the trail for dissemination of evidence-based practices for youth: Flexibility within fidelity. *Professional Psychology: Research and Practice, 38*(1), 13–20. https://doi.org/10.1037/0735-7028.38.1.13

Kendall, P. C., & Frank, H. E. (2018). Implementing evidence-based treatment protocols: Flexibility within fidelity. *Clinical Psychology: Science and Practice, 25*(4), Article e12271. https://doi.org/10.1111/cpsp.12271

Kiesler, D. J. (1992). Interpersonal Circle inventories: Pantheoretical applications to psychotherapy research and practice. *Journal of Psychotherapy Integration, 2*(2), 77–99. https://doi.org/10.1037/h0101246

Kiesler, D. J. (1996). *Contemporary interpersonal theory and research: Personality, psychopathology, and psychotherapy.* John Wiley & Sons.

Kiesler, D. J., & Watkins, L. M. (1989). Interpersonal complementarity and the therapeutic alliance: A study of the relationship in psychotherapy. *Psychotherapy, 26*(2), 183–194. https://doi.org/10.1037/h0085418

Klerman, G. L., Weissman, M. M., Rounsaville, B., & Chevron, E. S. (1984). *Interpersonal psychotherapy of depression.* Basic Books.

Koziol, L. F., & Budding, D. E. (2012). Procedural learning. In N. M. Seel (Ed.), *Encyclopedia of the sciences of learning* (pp. 2694–2696). Springer. https://doi.org/10.1007/978-1-4419-1428-6_670

Kupfer, D. J., Frank, E., Perel, J. M., Cornes, C., Mallinger, A. G., Thase, M. E., McEachran, A. B., & Grochocinski, V. J. (1992). Five-year outcome for maintenance therapies in recurrent depression. *Archives of General Psychiatry, 49*(10), 769–773. https://doi.org/10.1001/archpsyc.1992.01820100013002

Lambert, M. J. (2010). Yes, it is time for clinicians to monitor treatment outcome. In B. L. Duncan, S. C. Miller, B. E. Wampold, & M. A. Hubble (Eds.), *The heart and soul of change: Delivering what works in therapy* (2nd ed., pp. 239–266). American Psychological Association. https://doi.org/10.1037/12075-008

Linardon, J., Fitzsimmons-Craft, E. E., Brennan, L., Barillaro, M., & Wilfley, D. E. (2019). Dropout from interpersonal psychotherapy for mental health disorders: A systematic review and meta-analysis. *Psychotherapy Research, 29*(7), 870–881. https://doi.org/10.1080/10503307.2018.1497215

Markman, K. D., & Tetlock, P. E. (2000). Accountability and close-call counterfactuals: The loser who nearly won and the winner who nearly lost. *Personality and Social Psychology Bulletin, 26*(10), 1213–1224. https://doi.org/10.1177/0146167200262004

Markowitz, J. C., Lipsitz, J., & Milrod, B. L. (2014). Critical review of outcome research on interpersonal psychotherapy for anxiety disorders. *Depression and Anxiety, 31*(4), 316–325. https://doi.org/10.1002/da.22238

Markowitz, J. C., & Weissman, M. M. (2012). Interpersonal psychotherapy: Past, present and future. *Clinical Psychology & Psychotherapy, 19*(2), 99–105. https://doi.org/10.1002/cpp.1774

McAlpine, R., & Hillin, A. (2021). *Interpersonal psychotherapy for adolescents: A clinician's guide*. Taylor & Francis.

McGaghie, W. C., Issenberg, S. B., Barsuk, J. H., & Wayne, D. B. (2014). A critical review of simulation-based mastery learning with translational outcomes. *Medical Education, 48*(4), 375–385. https://doi.org/10.1111/medu.12391

McLeod, J. (2017). Qualitative methods for routine outcome measurement. In T. G. Rousmaniere, R. Goodyear, D. D. Miller, & B. E. Wampold (Eds.), *The cycle of excellence: Using deliberate practice to improve supervision and training* (pp. 99–122). Wiley Blackwell. https://doi.org/10.1002/9781119165590.ch5

Mennen, F. E., Palmer Molina, A., Monro, W. L., Duan, L., Stuart, S., & Sosna, T. (2021). Effectiveness of an interpersonal psychotherapy (IPT) group depression treatment for Head Start mothers: A cluster-randomized controlled trial. *Journal of Affective Disorders, 280*(Pt. B), 39–48. https://doi.org/10.1016/j.jad.2020.11.074

Miniati, M., Callari, A., Maglio, A., & Calugi, S. (2018). Interpersonal psychotherapy for eating disorders: Current perspectives. *Psychology Research and Behavior Management, 11*, 353–369. https://doi.org/10.2147/PRBM.S120584

Mulcahy, R., Reay, R. E., Wilkinson, R. B., & Owen, C. (2010). A randomised control trial for the effectiveness of group interpersonal psychotherapy for postnatal depression. *Archives of Women's Mental Health, 13*(2), 125–139. https://doi.org/10.1007/s00737-009-0101-6

Mychailyszyn, M. P., & Elson, D. M. (2018). Working through the blues: A meta-analysis on Interpersonal psychotherapy for depressed adolescents (IPT-A). *Children and Youth Services Review, 87*, 123–129. https://doi.org/10.1016/j.childyouth.2018.02.011

Norcross, J. C., & Guy, J. D. (2005). The prevalence and parameters of personal therapy in the United States. In J. D. Geller, J. C. Norcross, & D. E. Orlinsky (Eds.), *The psychotherapist's own psychotherapy: Patient and clinician perspectives* (pp. 165–176). Oxford University Press.

Norcross, J. C., Lambert, M. J., & Wampold, B. E. (2019). *Psychotherapy relationships that work* (3rd ed.). Oxford University Press.

O'Hara, M. W., Stuart, S., Gorman, L. L., & Wenzel, A. (2000). Efficacy of interpersonal psychotherapy for postpartum depression. *Archives of General Psychiatry, 57*(11), 1039–1045. https://doi.org/10.1001/archpsyc.57.11.1039

Orlinsky, D. E., & Rønnestad, M. H., & Collaborative Research Network of the Society for Psychotherapy Research. (2005). *How psychotherapists develop: A study of therapeutic work and professional growth*. American Psychological Association. https://doi.org/10.1037/11157-000

Owen, J., & Hilsenroth, M. J. (2014). Treatment adherence: The importance of therapist flexibility in relation to therapy outcomes. *Journal of Counseling Psychology, 61*(2), 280–288. https://doi.org/10.1037/a0035753

Pessagno, R. A. (2013). Using short-term group psychotherapy as an evidence-based intervention for first-time mothers at risk for postpartum depression *Perspectives in Psychiatric Care, 49*(3), 202–209. https://doi.org/10.1111/j.1744-6163.2012.00350.x

Prescott, D. S., Maeschalck, C. L., & Miller, S. D. (Eds.). (2017). *Feedback-informed treatment in clinical practice: Reaching for excellence*. American Psychological Association. https://doi.org/10.1037/0000039-000

Pu, J., Zhou, X., Liu, L., Zhang, Y., Yang, L., Yuan, S., Zhang, H., Han, Y., Zou, D., & Xie, P. (2017). Efficacy and acceptability of interpersonal psychotherapy for depression in adolescents:

A meta-analysis of randomized controlled trials. *Psychiatry Research*, *253*, 226–232. https://doi.org/10.1016/j.psychres.2017.03.023

Ravitz, P., Maunder, R., & McBride, C. (2008). Attachment, contemporary interpersonal theory and IPT: An integration of theoretical, clinical, and empirical perspectives. *Journal of Contemporary Psychotherapy*, *38*(1), 11–22. https://doi.org/10.1007/s10879-007-9064-y

Ravitz, P., Watson, P., Lawson, A., Constantino, M. J., Bernecker, S., Park, J., & Swartz, H. A. (2019). Interpersonal psychotherapy: A scoping review and historical perspective. *Harvard Review of Psychiatry*, *27*(3), 165–180. https://doi.org/10.1097/HRP.0000000000000219

Reay, R. E., Mulcahy, R., Wilkinson, R. B., Owen, C., Shadbolt, B., & Raphael, B. (2012). The development and content of an interpersonal psychotherapy group for postnatal depression. *International Journal of Group Psychotherapy*, *62*(2), 221–251. https://doi.org/10.1521/ijgp.2012.62.2.221

Reynolds, C. F., III, Dew, M. A., Martire, L. M., Miller, M. D., Cyranowski, J. M., Lenze, E., Whyte, E. M., Mulsant, B. H., Pollock, B. G., Karp, J. F., Gildengers, A., Szanto, K., Dombrovski, A. Y., Andreescu, C., Butters, M. A., Morse, J. Q., Houck, P. R., Bensasi, S., Mazumdar, S., . . . Frank, E. (2010). Treating depression to remission in older adults: A controlled evaluation of combined escitalopram with interpersonal psychotherapy versus escitalopram with depression care management. *International Journal of Geriatric Psychiatry*, *25*(11), 1134–1141. https://doi.org/10.1002/gps.2443

Reynolds, C. F., III, Frank, E., Perel, J. M., Imber, S. D., Cornes, C., Morycz, R. K., Mazumdar, S., Miller, M. D., Pollock, B. G., Rifai, A. H., Stack, J. A., George, C. J., Housck, P. R., & Kupfer, D. J. (1992). Combined pharmacotherapy and psychotherapy in the acute and continuation treatment of elderly patients with recurrent major depression: A preliminary report. *The American Journal of Psychiatry*, *149*(12), 1687–1692. https://doi.org/10.1176/ajp.149.12.1687

Reynolds, C. F., III, Miller, M. D., Pasternak, R. E., Frank, E., Perel, J. M., Cornes, C., Houck, P. R., Mazumdar, S., Dew, M. A., & Kupfer, D. J. (1999). Treatment of bereavement-related major depressive episodes in later life: A controlled study of acute and continuation treatment with nortriptyline and interpersonal psychotherapy. *The American Journal of Psychiatry*, *156*(2), 202–208. https://doi.org/10.1176/ajp.156.2.202

Rogers, C. R. (1957). The necessary and sufficient conditions of therapeutic personality change. *Journal of Consulting Psychology*, *21*(2), 95–103. https://doi.org/10.1037/h0045357

Rousmaniere, T. G. (2016). *Deliberate practice for psychotherapists: A guide to improving clinical effectiveness*. Routledge Press/Taylor & Francis. https://doi.org/10.4324/9781315472256

Rousmaniere, T. G. (2019). *Mastering the inner skills of psychotherapy: A deliberate practice handbook*. Gold Lantern Press.

Rousmaniere, T. G., Goodyear, R., Miller, S. D., & Wampold, B. E. (Eds.). (2017). *The cycle of excellence. Using deliberate practice to improve supervision and training*. Wiley Blackwell. https://doi.org/10.1002/9781119165590

Schultz, J., & Stuart, S. (2014). Interpersonal psychotherapy: A culturally adaptive treatment. *Psychotherapy in Australia*, *21*(1), 12–20.

Sockol, L. E. (2018). A systematic review and meta-analysis of interpersonal psychotherapy for perinatal women. *Journal of Affective Disorders*, *232*, 316–328. https://doi.org/10.1016/j.jad.2018.01.018

Sockol, L. E., Epperson, C. N., & Barber, J. P. (2011). A meta-analysis of treatments for perinatal depression. *Clinical Psychology Review*, *31*(5), 839–849. https://doi.org/10.1016/j.cpr.2011.03.009

Squire, L. R. (2004). Memory systems of the brain: A brief history and current perspective. *Neurobiology of Learning and Memory*, *82*(3), 171–177. https://doi.org/10.1016/j.nlm.2004.06.005

Stiles, W. B., Honos-Webb, L., & Surko, M. (1998). Responsiveness in psychotherapy. *Clinical Psychology: Science and Practice*, *5*(4), 439–458. https://doi.org/10.1111/j.1468-2850.1998.tb00166.x

Stiles, W. B., & Horvath, A. O. (2017). Appropriate responsiveness as a contribution to therapist effects. In L. G. Castonguay & C. E. Hill (Eds.), *How and why are some therapists better than others? Understanding therapist effects* (pp. 71–84). American Psychological Association. https://doi.org/10.1037/0000034-005

Stuart, S. (2019). *Interpersonal psychotherapy: A clinician's guide* (3rd ed.). Taylor & Francis.

Stuart, S., Pereira, X. V., & Chung, J. P. Y. (2021). Transcultural adaptation of interpersonal psychotherapy in Asia. *Asia-Pacific Psychiatry*, *13*(1), e12439. https://doi.org/10.1111/appy.12439

Stuart, S., & Robertson, M. (2003). *Interpersonal psychotherapy: A clinician's guide*. Edward Arnold.

Stuart, S., & Robertson, M. (2012). *Interpersonal psychotherapy: A clinician's guide* (2nd ed.). Taylor and Francis.

Stuart, S., Schultz, J., Back-Price, A., Belik-Tuller, O., Stuart-Parrigon, K., Ashen, C., Fairhurst, S., Grause, A., & Brandon, A. (2017). *Interpersonal psychotherapy*. Scientific American Psychiatry.

Stuart, S., Schultz, J. M., Palmer Molina, A., & Siber-Sanderowitz, S. (in press). Interpersonal psychotherapy: A review of theory, history, and evidence of efficacy. *Psychodynamic Psychiatry*.

Sullivan, H. S. (1953). *The interpersonal theory of psychiatry*. W. W. Norton & Co.

Taylor, J. M., & Neimeyer, G. J. (2017). Lifelong professional improvement: The evolution of continuing education. In T. G. Rousmaniere, R. Goodyear, S. D. Miller, & B. Wampold (Eds.), *The cycle of excellence: Using deliberate practice to improve supervision and training* (pp. 219–248). Wiley Blackwell.

Tracey, T. J. G., Wampold, B. E., Goodyear, R. K., & Lichtenberg, J. W. (2015). Improving expertise in psychotherapy. *Psychotherapy Bulletin*, *50*(1), 7–13.

Verdeli, H., Clougherty, K., Onyango, G., Lewandowski, E., Speelman, L., Betancourt, T. S., Neugebauer, R., Stein, T. R., & Bolton, P. (2008). Group interpersonal psychotherapy for depressed youth in IDP camps in northern Uganda: Adaptation and training. *Child and Adolescent Psychiatric Clinics of North America*, *17*(3), 605–624, ix. https://doi.org/10.1016/j.chc.2008.03.002

Wass, R., & Golding, C. (2014). Sharpening a tool for teaching: The zone of proximal development. *Teaching in Higher Education*, *19*(6), 671–684. https://doi.org/10.1080/13562517.2014.901958

Weissman, M. (2006). A brief history of interpersonal psychotherapy. *Psychiatric Annals*, *36*(8), 553–557.

Weissman, M. M., Markowitz, J. C., & Klerman, G. L. (2018). *The guide to interpersonal psychotherapy* (Updated and expanded ed.). Oxford University Press.

Zaretskii, V. (2009). The zone of proximal development: What Vygotsky did not have time to write. *Journal of Russian & East European Psychology*, *47*(6), 70–93. https://doi.org/10.2753/RPO1061-0405470604

Zhou, X., Hetrick, S. E., Cuijpers, P., Qin, B., Barth, J., Whittington, C. J., Cohen, D., Del Giovane, C., Liu, Y., Michael, K. D., Zhang, Y., Weisz, J. R., & Xie, P. (2015). Comparative efficacy and acceptability of psychotherapies for depression in children and adolescents: A systematic review and network meta-analysis. *World Psychiatry*, *14*(2), 207–222. https://doi.org/10.1002/wps.20217

Zhou, X., Teng, T., Zhang, Y., Del Giovane, C., Furukawa, T. A., Weisz, J. R., Li, X., Cuijpers, P., Coghill, D., Xiang, Y., Hetrick, S. E., Leucht, S., Qin, M., Barth, J., Ravindran, A. V., Yang, L., Curry, J., Fan, L., Silva, S. G., . . . Xie, P. (2020). Comparative efficacy and acceptability of antidepressants, psychotherapies, and their combination for acute treatment of children and adolescents with depressive disorder: A systematic review and network meta-analysis. *The Lancet Psychiatry*, *7*(7), 581–601. https://doi.org/10.1016/S2215-0366(20)30137-1

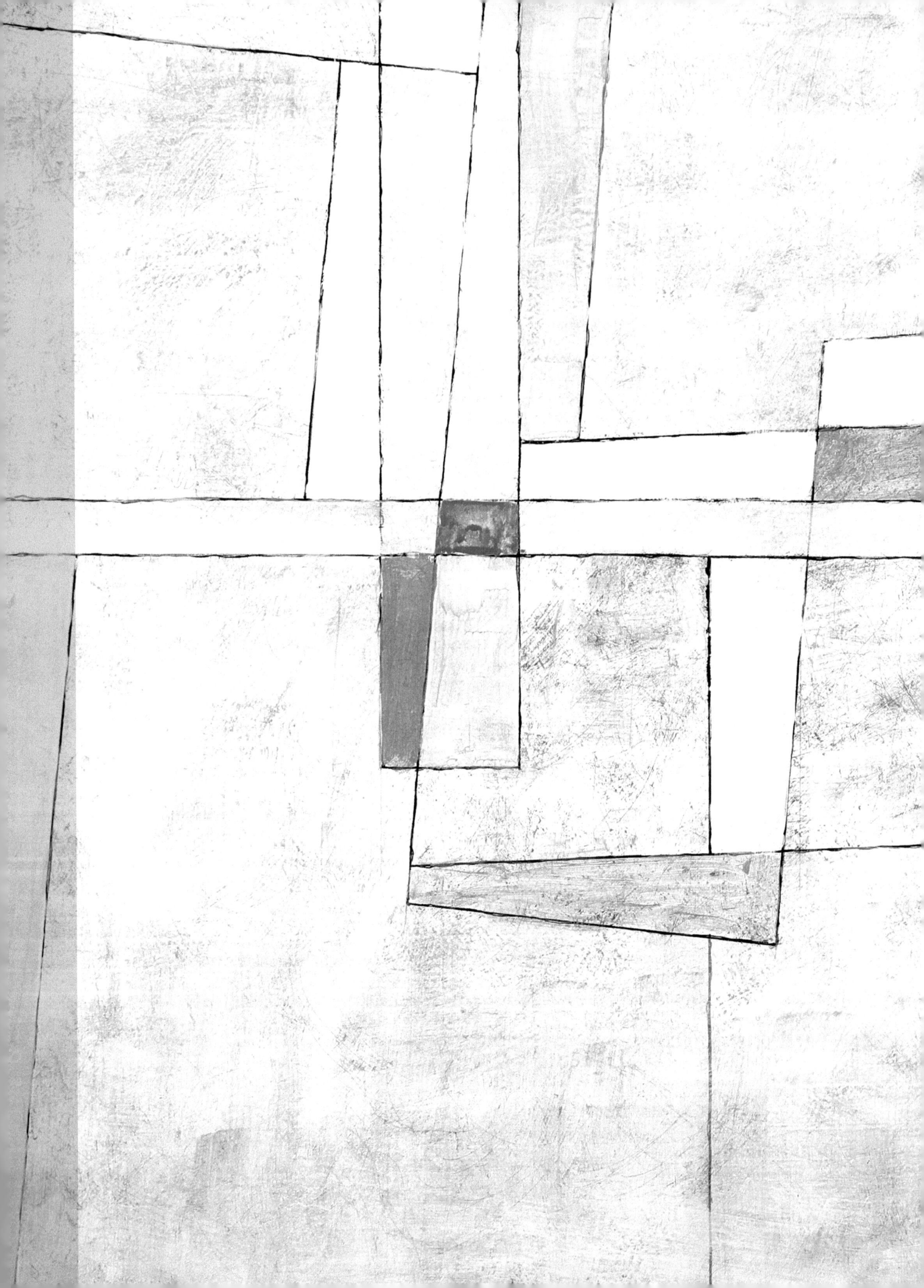

Index

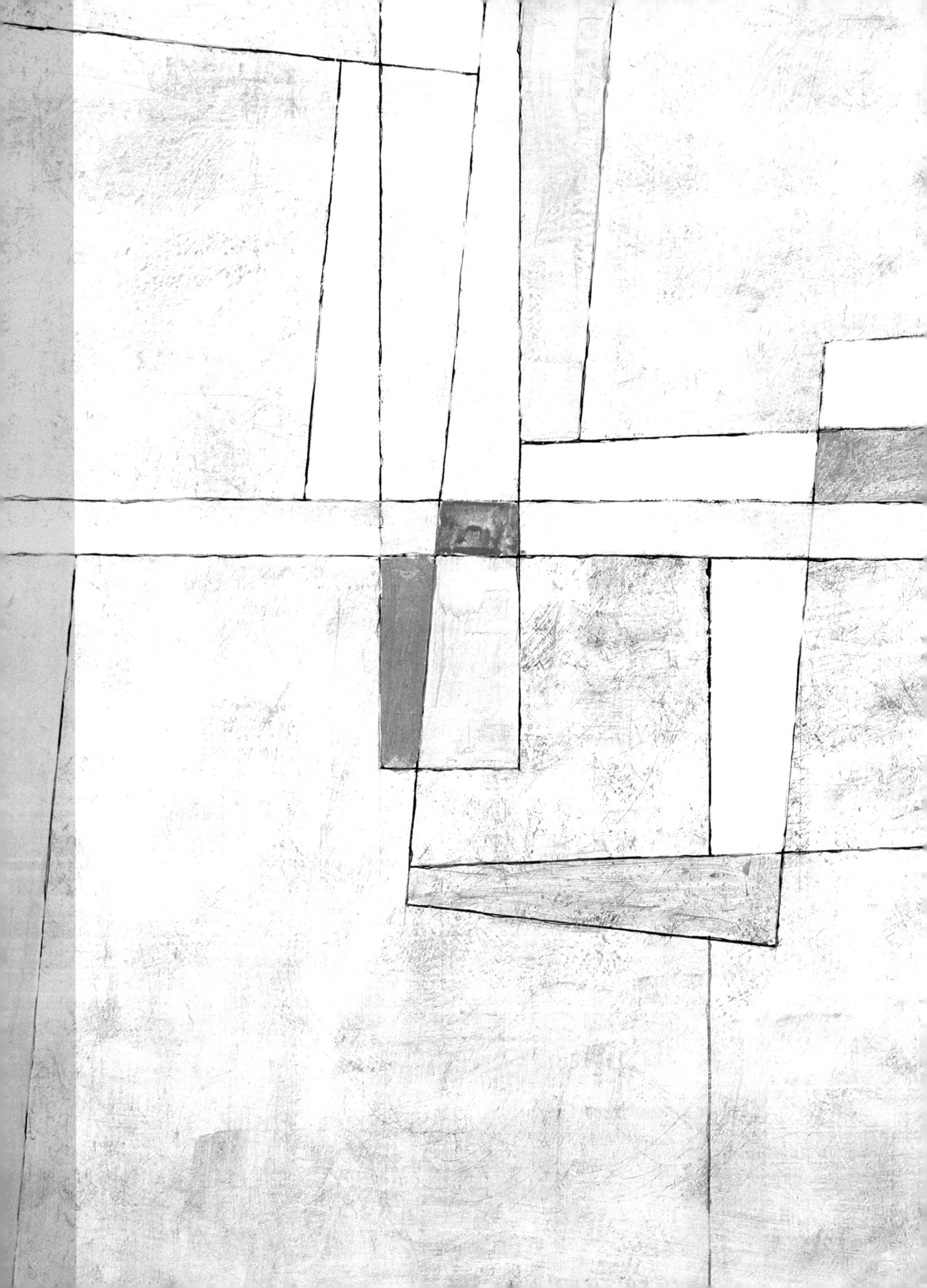

About the Authors

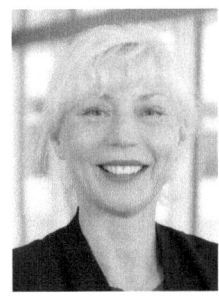

Olga Belik, PhD, is chief psychologist and senior director of training at the Providence Saint John's Health Center in Santa Monica, CA. She has been a fellow at the IPT Institute for more than a decade and provides national and international training, presentations, certifications, and consultations in interpersonal psychotherapy (IPT). She has coauthored articles related to IPT, clinical supervision, and training in supervision. Dr. Belik also serves on the board of directors of the California Psychological Association, Division II: Training and Education in Professional Psychology. In addition, she has maintained a forensic and consultative private practice for more than 20 years.

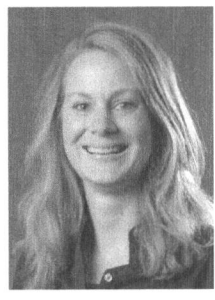

Jessica M. Schultz, PhD, is a licensed psychologist and professor of psychology at Augustana College (Rock Island, IL). She has been engaged in clinical work and research in interpersonal psychotherapy (IPT) for more than 15 years. Recognized as a fellow by the IPT Institute, her IPT training experience includes serving as a presenter, supervisor, and consultant for clinicians across the world. She coauthored the clinical guide *Interpersonal Psychotherapy: Clinician's Handbook* (IPT Institute Press) and multiple articles related to IPT. In addition to her academic and training roles, Dr. Schultz maintains a small clinical practice.

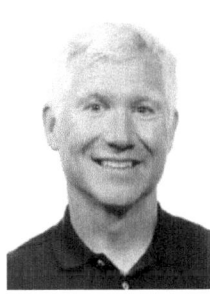

Scott Fairhurst, PhD, is a fellow at the IPT Institute, having first been certified as an interpersonal psychotherapy (IPT) clinician in 2016. He is the vice president of outcomes and evaluation, business analytics, and training at Pacific Clinics, a large behavioral health agency in California, where his work focuses on value-based care. Dr. Fairhurst's work is based on decades of clinical experience, primarily with clients whose mood and impulse difficulties tended to lead to dangerous situations. These situations were what first drew him to IPT, seeing the opportunities for progress in communication when there has been a pattern of escalation or harm.

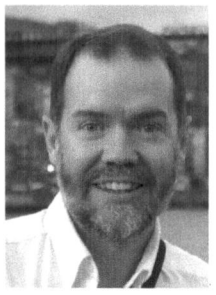

Scott Stuart, MD, is a psychiatrist and an emeritus professor in the Departments of Psychiatry, Psychology and Brain Sciences, Pediatrics, and Obstetrics and Gynecology at the University of Iowa (Iowa City, IA) and an adjunct clinical professor of psychiatry and behavioral sciences in the Keck School of Medicine at the University of Southern California, Los Angeles. He has been active in clinical work, education, and research in the areas of interpersonal psychotherapy (IPT) and perinatal psychiatry for over 3 decades.

Dr. Stuart is the founder and director of the IPT Institute. He has also authored over 100 chapters and articles on IPT and is the coauthor of *Interpersonal Psychotherapy: A Clinician's Guide* (2nd ed.), as well as the upcoming third edition, and IPT handbooks for adults, adolescents, and groups. He has been conducting workshops and training in IPT internationally for more than 30 years.

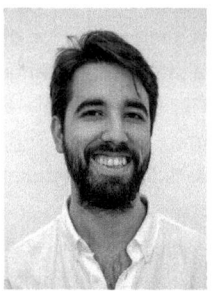

Alexandre Vaz, PhD, is cofounder and chief academic officer of Sentio University. He provides deliberate practice workshops and clinical training and supervision around the world. Dr. Vaz is the author or coeditor of many books on deliberate practice and psychotherapy training and two book series: Essentials of Deliberate Practice (American Psychological Association) and Advanced Therapeutics, Clinical and Interpersonal Skills (Elsevier). He has held multiple committee roles for the Society for the Exploration of Psychotherapy Integration and the Society for Psychotherapy Research. Dr. Vaz is founder and host of "Psychotherapy Expert Talks," an acclaimed interview series with distinguished psychotherapists and researchers.

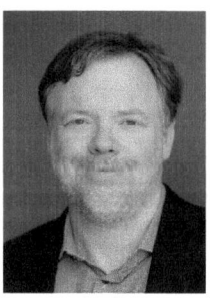

Tony Rousmaniere, PsyD, is cofounder and program director of Sentio University. He provides workshops, webinars, and clinical training and supervision around the world. He is the author or coeditor of many books on deliberate practice and psychotherapy training and two book series: Essentials of Deliberate Practice (American Psychological Association [APA]) and Advanced Therapeutics, Clinical and Interpersonal Skills (Elsevier). In 2017, he published the widely cited article "What Your Therapist Doesn't Know" in *The Atlantic*. Dr. Rousmaniere supports the open-data movement and publishes clinical outcome data on his website (https://www.drtonyr.com). He was awarded the Early Career Award by the Society for the Advancement of Psychotherapy (APA Division 29).